TUPORG

The *Unauthorized* Psychoanalysis Of Rudolph Giuliani:

The Zero of Ground Zero

Third Edition

James C. McIntosh, M.D.

CEMOTAP PUBLICATIONS

ISBN:978-0-9795972-0-6

Dedication: This Book is dedicated to and in memory of my father Van Little, Dr. Amos Wilson, Sister Abiola Sinclair and to my living heroes, Imhotep Gary Byrd, Queen Idia and all who have set the example.

Notice

These articles represent a combination of the unedited versions of articles that appeared in the Black Press between the years 1991 to 2002. Seven of these articles appeared during the seven-week period between March 28, 2000 And May 12, 2000 in a series called "The Unauthorized Psychoanalysis of Rudolph Giuliani. All seven stories were run nearly in their entirety in the Daily Challenge, The Amsterdam News and The Cemotap Drum. Several have also appeared at the website of The Black World Today. Com.

Acknowledgements

I thank The Creator for the members of my immediate family and my extended families of CEMOTAP, Committee to Eliminate Media Offensive to African People, U.A.M., United African Movement, NAN, National Action Network, MMWCCQ, Million Man and Woman Coordinating Committee Of Queens, Black Family Collective and The Nation Of Islam Mosque # 7C. Also, I give thanks for Professor Walter Bowe, Dr. Moses Powell, Shihan Ernest Miles, Shihan Ron Brabham, Professor Ronald (Smiley) Smith-Bey, Professor Pedro and everyone at Bedford Stuyvesant School of Martial Arts, (Sanuces Ryu.) All of these great men and women played a vital and positive role in my completing this book.

Also, I give special thanks to The Creator for the assistance of Amsterdam News Publisher Emeritus, Wilbert Tatum and Publisher, Elinor Tatum who have been relentless in their exposure of Rudolph Giuliani. Thanks for Idia (Betty Dopson), Editor of the CEMOTAP Drum, Tommy Watkins, Publisher of the Daily Challenge, Dawad Phillip, Editor of the Daily Challenge, and Herb Boyd, author and educator who gave access to their publications when others would not.

Table of Contents

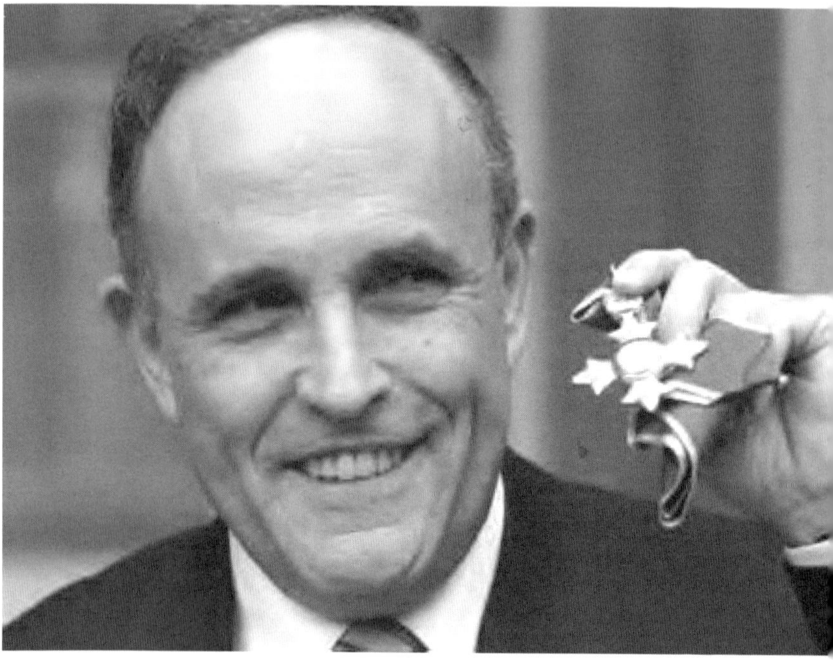

Chapter 1

Quotation: *"Power is the ability to define reality and have others respond to it as if it were their own."* ***Wade Noble***

"The Unauthorized Psychoanalysis of New York City Mayor, Rudolph Giuliani"

Reverend Al Sharpton demonstrated for the world last weekend just how many ordinary people are beginning to see that there is something wrong with Mayor Rudolph Giuliani. It happened at an awards program Saturday night, March 25, 2000 hosted by the Women's Auxiliary of National Action Network. Sharpton was in the process of giving an award to a woman with a background in psychology. Without batting an eye, Sharpton looked out at the audience where I was sitting and with a comedian's timing wondered aloud if I, (Dr. McIntosh), could help Rudy Giuliani. I'm

a psychiatrist, so I certainly do not regard mental illness as a joke. But not only did I howl, the entire audience howled in laughter. This reaction of these Patrick Dorismond sympathizers may just be the most reliable sign of how crazy the average person thinks Rudy is. (Patrick Dorismond was one of the unarmed private police officers hired by the businesses in the Madison Square Garden area of New York. Such officers are commonly called radio cops because of the large radio they wear on their belt in the spot where ordinary cops have guns. Dorismond had stopped after work at a bar in downtown New York to have a drink when an undercover cop approached him and asked if he knew where drugs might be purchased. Dorismond told the cop no. Somehow a few seconds later the cop shot Dorismond to death, the cop said by accident. In the hours after Dorismond's death the Giuliani public relations team decided to trash Dorismond and somehow justify the killing rather than apologize. In doing so Giuliani dredged up the sealed juvenile records of the minor misdeeds of Dorismund when he was in his early teens. Giuliani was harshly criticized by the victim's family, community leaders and even some of the more humane members of the New York tabloid press for exposing Dorismond's confidential childhood records. Characteristically Giuliani was unrepentant and publicly rationalized that the right to confidentiality ended with a person's death. Needless to say this was about the least consoling thing anyone could recall ever being said to the family of a law abiding victim of an admittedly accidental shooting.

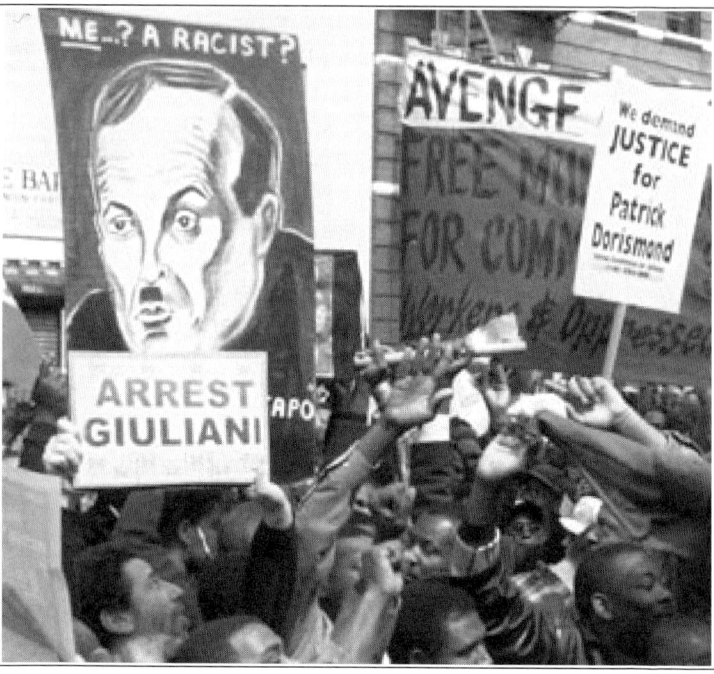
ME..? A RACIST?
ARREST GIULIANI
AVENGE
We demand JUSTICE for Patrick Dorismond

The Funeral of Patrick Dorismond

Laughter In The Face Of Terror

People at the event were still upset about the police foray into the Dorismond funeral procession earlier in the day. Clearly, no one thought that the disrespect Giuliani showed by sending so many police, including riot police to the funeral, was funny. Nor did anyone think the Mayor's boycott of the funeral or the words of condemnation he had uttered about the victim of a murder the police themselves have termed an accident.

Rather, the crowd was releasing the tension caused by the incongruity between the reality of the ever-growing list of unarmed Black men being killed by the police and the behavior, speech and implied underlying thinking of Rudolph Giuliani. After all, Giuliani is supposed to be the mayor representing all the people of the city, including those who have been killed and their families. If it weren't such a matter of life and death, the mayor's statements and actions regarding Patrick Dorismond would be hilarious at face value. The mayor's position has essentially been," What's all the hubbub about? A good cop says it was an accident and besides - Look right here. This sealed juvenile record clearly indicates that at age 13 it was apparent that this person was going to grow up to be someone likely to masquerade as a hardworking family man in the field of law enforcement, pretending just to be standing on the street, but actually doing so just for the purpose of harassing the cops."

Giuliani's absolutely straight face, complete with an indignant scowl, is what caps it all. People from across the political spectrum are noticing what I believe any psychiatrically trained person could have told them all along - something is wrong with the mayor.

Et Tu Bratton

Reverend Jesse Jackson characterized the mayor's response to police shootings of unarmed Black men as "more mental" than mean. Even the mayor's own ex-police chief was moved to imply last week that the mayor is psychotic. Said William Bratton, with a phrase that could just as easily been uttered about himself, the mayor is "off of the reservation. He's beating the drum before the guy has even been laid in the ground."

For years, mayoral critics, such as New York Newsday columnist Jimmy Breslin, as well as a few others, have said the mayor is paranoid. Now, however, even former Giuliani supporters such as former mayor, Ed Koch and Reverend Floyd Flake, pastor, Allen AME Church, Jamaica, New York have said similar things. Reverend Floyd Flake was moved a few weeks ago to use the words, "paranoid schizophrenic" and "megalomaniac" in reference to the mayor. I wouldn't want to stake my professional license on it, but in my opinion all these descriptions, while in the ballpark actually miss the mark. The mayor does have a problem, but each of his critics describes just one aspect of his problem, much in the manner of the proverbial blind men who each describe an elephant based on the part each has encountered. Resulting in separate descriptions of the elephant as like a wall, like roman columns and like a snake.

Rudy Is More Troubling Than Troubled

In my opinion, the mayor is actually not psychotic. I do not believe he has a biochemical imbalance that makes his mind play tricks on him. I similarly do not believe he is neurotic. He's not a conflicted person plagued with anxiety or sad feelings. No, the mayor is more of a troubling person than a troubled person. He is not feeling stress like the people or the families of the people his words and actions hurt. In fact, the more he utters hurtful words and engages in the hurtful behavior that he is driven to engage in, the less stress he feels.

In my opinion, Rudy has a condition described in The American Psychiatric Association's Diagnostic and Statistical Manual IV as "Personality Disorder Not Otherwise Specified." This is a term usually used when a person manifests a character disorder that either doesn't just fit neatly into one of the more well known personality disorders such as Paranoid Personality, Obsessive Compulsive Personality, Histrionic Personality Disorder, Antisocial Personality Disorder and Narcissistic Personality Disorder. The term is also used when a person manifests a mixture of character traits from two or more of the common personality disorders.

In my opinion, Rudy is remarkable in that his words and actions since adulthood and his background prior to adulthood suggest he manifests enough pathological traits to essentially meet the criteria for all of the above named personality disorders.

Translation From Psychobabble To English

For those who prefer their analysis in plain English rather than Psychobabble: It is my assertion that Rudy's behavior and words suggest that he has a "self righteous, bull headed streak," an "overly suspicious streak," a 'dramatic exhibitionist streak," a " crooked and dishonest streak" and a " selfish, self-absorbed streak." In subsequent articles, I will document exactly which behaviors and statements led me to believe as I do. I will also explain the defense mechanisms associated with each of these character disorders or "streaks" and how they have manifested themselves in Rudy's behaviors and statements.I will further develop a formulation for what caused these distortions in Rudy's character and attempt to explain why he has chosen Blacks as his scapegoats and how and why he uses the defense mechanism "undoing" so frequently. Lastly, I will summarize his history and mental status and make my recommendations for his treatment. Will I mention the love roots of his racial obsessions, his incestuous past, the cause of his families' flight from Brooklyn, his cross dressing, his tavern owning parents, his Kennedy obsession, his alleged torture of an Auschwitz victim, his use of the police to intimidate his critics, his teen ideas of a hot date, and his exhibitionistic relationship with his tax subsidized lady friend? Yes, I will.Stay tuned! Buy every edition of the black Press so you won't miss a word or the very loud snap from inside the bonkers bunker.

On February 4,1999, one of the most Bizarre shootings in the history of New York occurred during the Giuliani Administration. An unarmed African Immigrant with no criminal record was murdered on his door step by several police officers who fired a total of 41 or more shots at him with at least 18 striking him. The officers defense was that Mr. Diallo had reached in his pocket for something, the press accepted this explanation and_ speculated that Mr. Diallo had reached possibly for a wallet. Remarkably, the courts cleared the officers of all charges in February of 2000. The meeting mentioned in the beginning of this chapter occurred on the one year anniversary of the cops initial indictment by a grand jury. It was a meeting to organize a city wide boycott of white business in protest of the gross injustice represented by this case.

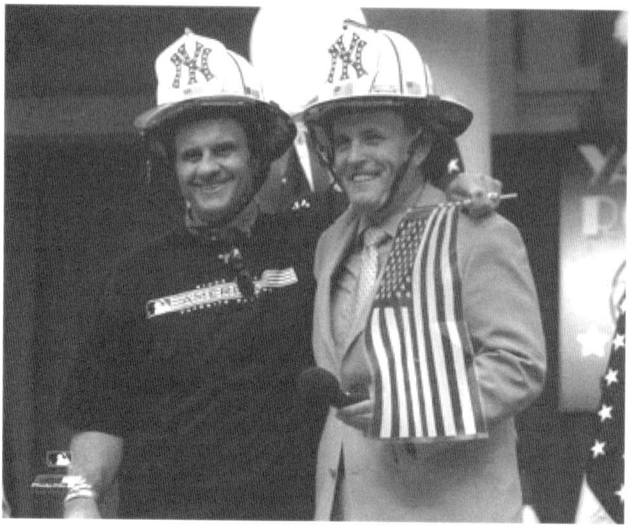

Quotation: "*Power is the ability to reward our friends and punish our enemies.*" ***Maulana Karenga***

Chapter 2

Psycho-Rudy Must Be Held Accountable

At a packed citywide meeting of the newly formed Amadou Diallo Coalition at Maranatha Baptist Church on March 31, 2000, last Thursday, in Jamaica Queens, Attorney Alton Maddox, Jr. made an offhand, perhaps, facetious remark regarding the mayor's mental state. Perhaps thinking ahead to a future War Crimes Tribunal, Maddox said, "We don't want to make him (label him) insane. We want him to be accountable for his wrongs."

Mayor Giuliani out of focus.

It is in that spirit and in keeping with those instructions that this second installment of my 101% objective, but thoroughly unauthorized psychoanalysis from afar is written. The mayor is indeed accountable for all that he has done. To review my contentions thus far, Giuliani is not psychotic. He has not, in a formal sense, lost contact with reality. In those instances where he appears to have done so, he is, in my opinion, not hallucinating, but simply telling a balding if not bald-faced lie. For example, back in 1982 when he was the Justice Department official in charge of the Immigration and Naturalization Service, he—as part of establishing a rationale for keeping Haitian Refugees locked in detention camps—claimed to have seen no evidence of political repression during a visit to Haiti. In the land of the Ton Ton Macoutes, he claimed to have seen police in "extremely light" amounts.

He followed this infamous report in 1982 with an interview in Barron's financial magazine in 1983. In this interview he claimed that the male Haitian detainees had to be separated from the females because the men would rape them. His exact words were, "And the women get very upset, because if you let the men into the women's camp, they go around raping them. So you have to separate them."

A Bald Faced Lie Does Not an Hallucination Make

Yet in 1989, several INS officials denied that any such rapes ever occurred. Maria Lula Rodrigues, a former U.S. Public Health Office screening officer, said, "The women did not get upset because they were getting raped. I was there from the beginning and I don't remember any such episodes." Greg Leo, the director of Congressional and Public Affairs of the Immigration Service was quoted as saying the agency "had not turned up any records of alleged rapes." Also by 1989, Giuliani was claiming he hadn't been fooled a bit in Haiti. His exact words were, "I didn't come away from it with the notion that there was no political repression in Haiti." In instances like this, Giuliani is not hallucinating. He's simply grasping at straws and fabricating a web from those he catches. Neither is Giuliani neurotic; he is not generally suffering from internal conflicts. He only suffers when he is punished for carrying out his hurtful policies and uttering his hurtful words. Giuliani fits the description of a person having what is called simply a personality disorder.

Exactly Which Kind Of Loony Is Rudy?

In my opinion, the American Psychiatric Association's description of "Personality Disorder Not Otherwise Specified" fits him best, in that he seems to have traits from five specific personality disorders. I will discuss the thread and the glue that holds these traits together. For indeed, it is not any single one or two traits that make the mayor obnoxious, rather it is the way these traits seem to work together that make him the difficult and unlikable person that he is. In my opinion, Rudy elects to do and say the things he does because these repugnant actions and words make him feel better, even as they make others feel worse. Many people have called him "loony" for this. But it's important to specify just which kind of "loony," in case, as Maddox suggests, he can ever be brought to trial. The mayor takes precautions, however, against this ever happening

Rudy-centric Thinking

Like all successful dictators and most paranoids, the mayor is monumentally hyper-vigilant. This is perhaps best symbolized by his multimillion-dollar bunker and his barricaded City Hall. This hyper-vigilance, plus his tendency to project and personalize, has led many to call him simply paranoid. However, there is a quality that links this paranoid tendency to four other personality disorders whose most obnoxious characteristics wed to shape the personality of Rudolph Giuliani. That quality is self-centeredness. This self-centeredness manifests itself even in the obsessive compulsive component of his personality, in the sense that such character disordered people cannot delegate tasks unless the person to whom they delegate is willing to perform the tasks in exactly the manner the obsessive has instructed. Ask ex-school chancellors Ramon Cortines and Rudy Crew about that. Mayor Rudy booted them out the second they wouldn't walk exactly in the dance steps he had painted on the floor. That is the nature of the self-centered obsessive.

Entitled Arrogance and a Lack Of Empathy

Narcissistic people, on the other hand, are self-centered in an entirely different manner. Narcissists believe they are special people entitled to special treatment. They often show arrogant haughty attitudes and exhibit a singular lack of empathy. The mayor, who until last year's mass arrests for civil disobedience temporarily half-opened his eyes, arrogantly felt he could simply refuse to talk to the city's Black elected officials, including State Comptroller Carl McCall, with whom he did not speak for four years. Giuliani had even refused to admit entry to auditors sent to city offices by McCall. Giuliani put the A in arrogance.

How about empathy? Giuliani once had an absolutely astounding phone conversation with a grieving mother on his radio talk show on Radio WNYC. The woman, Margarita Rosario, was confronting the mayor on the fact that two of his former bodyguards, New York City Detectives Patrick Brosnan, and James Crowe, had shot her son and two companions a total of 22 times in the back and sides. Mrs. Rosario said her son had no criminal record. Instead of offering sympathy the mayor called her son a criminal and on the air said, "Maybe you should ask yourself some questions about the way he was brought up and the things that happened to him." That's certainly close to zero on the empathy meter.

Chinatown Hysteria

This example of popping off to a grieving mother also exhibits some of the impulsivity that can be attributed to the component responsible for a third source of Giuliani's self-centeredness. That component is his histrionic component, (formerly called hysterical). It's the set of tendencies in Giuliani that makes him constantly seek to be the center of attention. If there is a newsworthy event, he wants to get into the act and even get credit for things he has had little or nothing to do with. It's this tendency that in part caused him to develop a competitive antagonism with ex-police commissioner, William Bratton, somewhat of a ham himself who had his own press secretary, John Miller.

It is this histrionic component that contributes to Rudy's drive to dress up like Marilyn Monroe over and over. It is also perhaps what made him take a picture together dining with Christyne Lategano, a woman many, including the magazine *Vanity Fair*, have labeled as his mistress. According to an article by columnist and author, Jimmy Breslin, this picture hangs as a greeting to customers at a Chinese Restaurant along Broadway. Hysterics also are known to pick taboo love objects such as much younger women or cousins. Of course, it is also well documented that Giuliani was married for 14 years to Regina Peruggi, the daughter of his father's first cousin, Salvatore. But the topic is selfishness. What thread links Peruggi, Donna Hanover, Christyne Lategano and one other woman who will be discussed in more detail in a later article.

Criminal Minded

Yet another form of selfishness and self-centeredness is contributed by the mayor's antisocial personality component. Antisocial does not mean unsociable as is commonly thought, rather, it is the set of characteristics previously called sociopathic, psychopathic, or at one time, simply criminal characteristics. Antisocial characteristics are the type manifested by the chronic, habitual and flagrant disregard for the rights of others. Mark Green, the NYC Public Advocate, even prior to last week's 5.8 million dollar settlement with the Brooklyn Museum of Art estimated a five million dollar cost for the 22 "first amendment" and "freedom of information" cases Giuliani was litigating at taxpayers expense. Giuliani even flagrantly disregards the rights of people who have been friendly to him such as the Daily News Newspaper administrators who had to take him to court to gain access to information regarding subway crime figures.

Access to such information was not only considered a right, but prior to Giuliani's reign, was considered to be commonplace and routine. Just last week, Judge Guido Calabrese lambasted Giuliani in a 63-page ruling citing 18 cases of Giuliani's assault on the first amendment rights of the citizens of New York. In all of these cases, judges had to force Giuliani to honor these rights. Although Calabrese was ruling in the case of photographer Spencer Tunick, the same tendency to disregard the rights of others is equally well-illustrated by the case of Chris Ofili. Ofili is the artist whose painting of a Black Madonna using dung as one of his materials, infuriated the Mayor. The mayor was so infuriated, in fact, that he attempted to cut the funding of the Brooklyn Museum of Art which dared to exhibit the paintings against his wishes. Although the same antisocial characteristics are exhibited in this instance, the case is also illustrative of Rudy's paranoid component.

Rudy Chewing Dung

The best description of the paranoid I ever read was contained not in a medical journal or a psychiatric textbook, but in Mad Magazine 40 years ago. (If the originators of this magazine could have known the mayor, they might have named it Giuliani Magazine.) Mad magazine defined a paranoid as a person who walks down the street steps on a piece of gum and says, "How did they know I was going to take this route today?" In that last sentence just substitute the words "in a museum" for "down the street" and "dung" for "gum" and you can see Giuliani. He saw Ofili's painting, which was simply Ofili's expression, as a personal attack on his religion. An unwarranted sense of persecution, use of the mental processes, projection and personalization are three hallmarks of the paranoid. These primitive mental processes permeate both the mayor's personal style and administration. They are the characteristics that make him seem most crazy to others and most sane to himself. They are also the characteristics that make him most scary to others. In fact, some textbooks cover the homicidal patient as a subchapter of the paranoid patient.

It's Not Easy Being Mean

(When a friend of mine read the first installation of this series, he called a mutual friend. He asked, "what Is James trying to do, get himself shot?" He was not speaking figuratively.) Paranoids are classically quite vindictive, and you can never put anything past them. Rudy's selective prosecution and persecution of enemies real and imagined has been legendary. One elected official was threatened with a homeless shelter being built in his neighborhood because of his opposition to some policy of the mayor. One of my sources tells me that there are those who even believed that a break-in that occurred at the home of one of the mayor's cousins was quite suspicious. What was so suspicious was that whoever broke into the home took the time to overturn an urn of ashes of the mayor's former wife and cousin's deceased Black companion. But that is the subject of another article. The incidents of paranoid vindictiveness that I would like to speculate on right now are closer to my own home than the mayor's ex wife, cousin, wife, cousin, slap, Chinatown.

Rudy's Troopers Terrorized My Home

A few years ago I wrote a number of articles critical of Mayor Giuliani and a couple of his radio pals, Jay Diamond and Bob Grant. Giuliani appeared on their WABC AM radio programs many times. Giuliani has actually appeared on shows where Bob Grant called for the drowning of Haitian refugees and once participated in a racial skit where Jay Diamond did a minstrel voice imitation of former Black Mayor David Dinkins. Both Diamond and Grant frequently referred to Dinkins as the washroom attendant.

Diamond whom I had helped to expose as a racist eventually became so enraged that he broadcast a mock bombing of me, the entire staff of a newspaper I wrote for, and members of CEMOTAP. He also alleged over the airwaves that I had a phony Medical Degree.

I sued him and WABC radio for slander. The law firm that defended Diamond and WABC when I sued them, was Giuliani's former firm. The judge that ruled that it was "ok" for Diamond to make such false statements was Judge Julius Vinik. It was an unusual enough decision to be covered in the New York Law Journal, since there are specific regulations on the books against slandering a licensed physician and surgeon (that's what my license says, physician and surgeon). What was also interesting was that in the over one and a half hours of taped excerpts of venom I had collected of Diamond criticizing and threatening me was a veiled threat of police perhaps being interested in me. Diamond does not control the police, but almost a year to the day after he uttered such threats, police came to my home. With guns drawn, they came into my back yard shouted "halt" to my adult developmentally disabled son.

I Ain't Mad - Rudy's Mad - I'm Just Righteously Angry

My son, not understanding anything except the gun, ran into the house. I was not home, and my son could only explain that men with drawn guns had chased him in the house. My wife who is an ex-Black Panther gathered my two youngest children up in her arms and fled with my older son through the front door to her father's house. When my father- in -law returned with my wife, the police were in my house explaining that they thought my son was a robber. It was broad daylight. He was our own driveway. Why didn't they chase him? Why didn't they arrest him? They did none of these things because their purpose was at that time only to intimidate.

Sometime later a car I was driving was towed from in front of my house in the early morning for being only 6 feet from a fire hydrant. There was not one outstanding ticket on this car at the time, but the car was not simply ticketed. It was, for no reason, towed. On many days when I would write stories about Giuliani and his buddies, our home newspaper would be delivered to my wife's job instead of our house.

Now, what is this last section all about? Am I saying the Mayor had anything to do with any of these things? Of course I believe he did. As the chief executive of the city, he is certainly responsible for the buck wild behavior of the police. If for nothing else, his appearances on the radio programs of Jay Diamond and Bob Grant created the climate for every one of the murders of unarmed Black men and the false arrests and harassment of his critics. If they can still blame Minister Farrakhan in the year 2000 for a climate 35 years ago, in a city he did not govern, then Giuliani can certainly be blamed for climate in the city he currently governs for the short but tumultuous period he has governed. The only difference is that Giuliani is knowingly and willingly, creating such a climate and is as guilty as sin for the climate he has created.

During last year's mass arrests several of the mayor's critics, including Carl McCall, New York State Comptroller, complained of being held in detention longer than the other demonstrators. At least two artists critical of the mayor say they have been arrested for it. Robert Lederman, who paints works depicting Giuliani as a Nazi, says he has been arrested over 40 times with each arrest resulting in a dismissal. What a waste of tax dollars and what vindictiveness! Even more alarming perhaps is the case of artist Steven Powers whose parody of Chris Ofili's painting "Sensation" called Doody Rudy, featured the mayor as a Madonna. An event was to be held where spectators were urged to toss fake elephant dung at the painting. Powers home was within days of the event invaded by police who found a pair of brass knuckles he used as a wall decoration and arrested him.

Did Jay Diamond and the mayor have anything to do with those police who invaded my home and made my wife and children flee into the winter streets in their stocking feet? I don't know. Am I saying that was an act of paranoid vindictiveness? Or worse, am I saying that this unauthorized psychoanalysis is revenge? Of course not, that would make me a paranoid and obviously I can't be paranoid. I'm a psychiatrist!

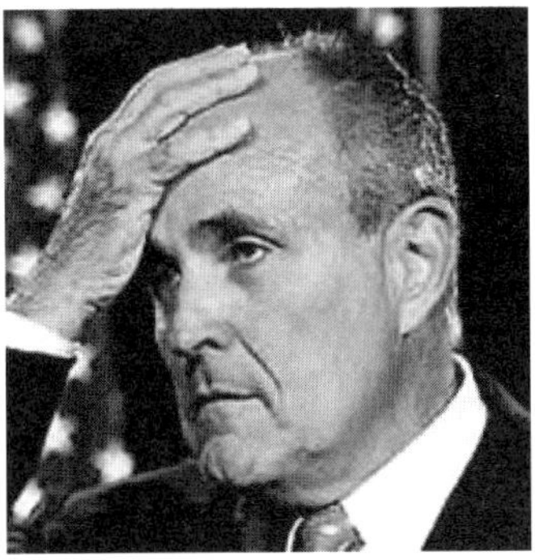

Quotation: *"If the enemy general is arrogant and obnoxious, provoke him.".* ***Sun Tzu***

Chapter 3

Free Association and That Other "N" Word

Freud popularized a technique called free association which has been the cornerstone of psychoanalysis, and the butt of the humor of countless comedians. The main idea in free association is that if a person says the first thing on their mind, freely without inhibition and these productions (words) are analyzed, unconscious thoughts will be unlocked. In one famous comedy routine, a white psychiatrist asks the patient Richard Prior to freely associate by saying the first word that comes into his mind. The process starts out benignly with the psychiatrist saying neutral words such as "dog," and Prior's calmly responding equally neutrally with words such as "cat." Ultimately, however, it ends with the psychiatrist saying some racially charged words and Prior's angrily responding with equally charged words, such as "honkey." When the psychiatrist finally says the "N" word, Prior attacks the psychiatrist screaming, "*Dead Honkey*," to gales of laughter from the audience. Strangely enough, when many New Yorkers "free associate" to the name Giuliani another "N" word crops up. That word is "Nazi."

The Right To Remain Silenced

A German artist by the name of Haacke is currently showing at the Whitney Museum until June. His exhibit features several of the mayor's more Nazi like statements that were uttered when he

sought to block artist Chris Ofili's painting, "Sensation," from being exhibited at the Brooklyn Museum of Art. Chris Ofili's use of dung as a medium in his painting of a Black Madonna was interpreted by the mayor as an attack on the Catholic Religion. One statement featured in the exhibit is the classic nazi like allegation that: "Civilization has been about trying to find the right place to put excrement, not on the walls of museums." The following Giuliani gems may or may not be in Haackes exhibit but they fully demonstrate the principle that if we interpret the free unfettered response of the patient we can get to the root of what is in their unconscious or hidden mind.

"Freedom is about Authority"- New York Times 3-17-94

"You don't have a right not to be identified"- New York Times 12-17-98

"An exhibition of paintings is not as communicative as speech or live entertainment, and the artists' constitutional interest is thus minimal" - A legal brief filed against street artists on Giuliani's behalf.

A Blitzkrieg on The Bill Of Rights

Many people, including the judges in at least 22 major first amendment and freedom of information cases, have wondered to which constitution Rudy was referring? For even the American constitution with all its flaws does have a so-called Bill of Rights. Giuliani has blitzed through this Bill of Rights like Hitler marching through Poland. Let me free-associate a bit.

The 1st Amendment - The 22 cases mentioned above. The 2nd Amendment (pertaining to the right to bear arms) - The infamous police street crimes unit and the police ***Operation Condor*** initiative have deprived people of the right to bear not only arms but wallets, beepers, keys and candy bars - having shot and or killed people allegedly for carrying any of these items.

The 3rd and 4th amendment (pertaining to the right of people to be free from soldiers or police camping in their homes or breaking into their homes for illegal searches) In May of 1998 Police threw a concussion grenade into the home of a Black man, Basil Shorter. For over an hour, Shorter his wife and 14-year-old developmentally disabled daughter were terrorized by police, camped in his home, ripping it apart looking for non-existent drugs. His naked daughter was actually snatched by police out of the shower. A similar attack under the pretense of searching the "wrong apartment" for drugs terrorized Asija Fulton and her 6-year-old son. Police with a battering ram charged in on them with guns drawn. One other case notable only for its being reported in the media involved Ellis Elliot, who had 22 shots fired through his front door by police, again at the wrong apartment searching for drugs. Precinct Chief Martin O'Boyle admitted to reporters in connection to the Basil Shorter case, that in 1997 out of approximately 2900 search warrants issued to police about 500 resulted in no contraband being found. Wrong apartment? Wrong country!

The 5th Amendment (pertaining to self-incrimination and private property not being seized without due process)- Giuliani's police, without the benefit of any amendments to the Bill of Rights, any jury or any judge, are seizing people's cars for anything from drugs to speeding. At one time there was even talk about seizing people's dogs.

Bells On Ze Bicycle Not In Ze Belfry

Police practice under Giuliani has resulted in numerous Black men engaged in no crime other than minor traffic infractions such as riding a bicycle without a bell being jailed- not ticketed, but jailed and sent through the system. Newsday reported in October of 1998 that a man named Anthony Williams spent over 20 hours in jail for this crime. Another named Willie Green did time for the same offense. Still another named Michael Martin was jailed for riding a bicycle with no taillight or headlight. Two women selling oranges were jailed for a whole day for obstructing traffic. These arrests all occurred in two precincts in Central Brooklyn where few whites live. A look at the other Constitutional amendments will reveal that about the only freedom Giuliani has been unable to curtail is the right of free association in the psychiatric sense.

Mr. Bill Tatum, Free Associates

It is perhaps for that reason that in the March 30 edition of The Amsterdam News, Chairman Emeritus Wilbert A. Tatum wrote "Hitler and Giuliani are Kindred Spirits." It is likewise in that same vein, perhaps, that ex-police Commissioner Bratton's press agent John Miller resigned in disgust over Giuliani's obsession with stopping leaks to the press and others by the police. When Giuliani ordered Miller to fire half his staff, Miller refused to be a loyal Nazi saying, "I'm loyal to the mayor...there were loyal Nazi's too... loyalty wears down."

Artist Robert Lederer, who paints Giuliani as a Nazi, has at last count been arrested 41 times with 41 failures to convict. Giuliani's response has been humorless and Nazi like. He was quoted in the New York Times of 3-28-99 as deadpanning, "The comparisons to Adolph Hitler and fascism have to stop." The question the free "associators" ask in response to Rudy's edict is the question that has infuriated dictators from time immemorial - Why?

Workfare Will Work You Free, Or At Least Cheap

If it looks, walks talks and oppresses like a Nazi, then call it a Nazi. A survivor of the Auschwitz death camp Simon Berger, took an ad in a Jewish newspaper called Algemeiner Journal back in 1989 that adds a more personal and direct basis for the repeated association of Giuliani with Nazi-philosophy and practice. Berger complained that when he was brought to Giuliani's U.S. Attorney's office in 1986, he was seated by federal agents in front of a blackboard with the words "Arbeit Macht Frei." The words mean, "Work Will Set You Free." They are the words that were posted at the front gate of that same infamous concentration camp where Berger had been imprisoned, Auschwitz.

Was the intent of Giuliani and/or his staff to induce the acute manifestations of Post Traumatic Stress Syndrome in Mr. Berger? Did lawman Giuliani and his staff think that this was a fair way to gather evidence in the criminal matter they were investigating? Did they feel it would perhaps crack the fortitude and break the will of Mr. Berger to resist.? If that was not Rudy's thinking, he couldn't have done a better imitation of a Nazi who was trying to do so. Ultimately, the blackboard incident was swept under the rug and termed a coincidence.

Any Resemblance To Anybody Wearing A Moustache Is Purely Coincidental

But, if during the course of my proposed therapy of Rudolph Giuliani, Rudy found himself sitting in front of a blackboard that said "James Hall, St. Philip Neri Church," I wonder if he would believe that was a coincidence. The St. Philip Neri Church is where Rudy married his second cousin, Regina, in 1968. James Hall is a Black man who will be spoken of in later articles whose involvement with Regina may allow us to interpret not only Rudy's attacks on Blacks, but also his attack on CUNY and remediation. But suffice it to say now that in the case of Berger, Rudy, as he did in the case of Regina in 1982 when he had the marriage annulled and denied any knowledge or culpability in the 14 year incestuous affair.

According to Attorney Barry Slotnick, in the Berger case Giuliani never took any fingerprints or handwriting samples to determine whom else if anyone in his office was to blame. This lapse is, of course, probably just another coincidence, a mental lapse in a man so suspicious and investigatively thorough that he obtains sealed juvenile arrest records of victims of, so called, accidental police killings as a basis for determining if he should send a sympathy cards to their families. This man with the temperament to obtain fingerprints from applicants for public assistance and DNA samples from alleged attempted jaywalkers forgot to take fingerprints or handwriting samples in a torture case. *That* is a coincidence.

However there are a few other coincidences in Rudy's history that make Tatum's comparison of Giuliani to Hitler so appropriate. Let's free-associate through a few.

Concentration Camps - Haitian Detention Camps

Luftwaffe – NYC Police strafe the Million Youth March

SS Unit - the SC Unit (Street Crimes Unit)

Arbeit Macht Frei - Workfare.

In yet another incident with this emphasis on work ethic, Jason Turner, Giuliani's Welfare commissioner was forced by Jewish groups in 1997 to apologize for using the phrase "Work Sets You Free" in describing Giuliani's workfare program. Adam Segall of the Anti Defamation League of B'nai B'rith said at the time regarding Jason Turner's perhaps Freudian Slip, "Obviously, Mr. Turner had heard this expression at another time and may have been ignorant of the context in which he heard it." Now who else could have used this phrase in Turner's presence? Everybody, let's count to 3 and Free associate. "Einz, zwei, drei - Rudy!"

Quotation: "When you become sentimental about power, you don't have it anymore.: **Dr. John Henrik Clarke**

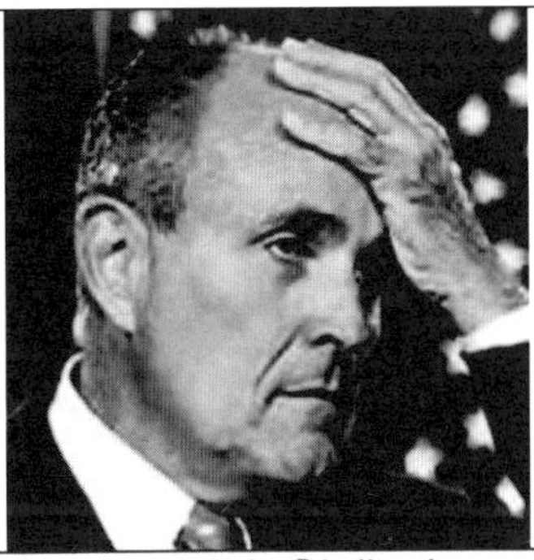

Rudolph Giuliani

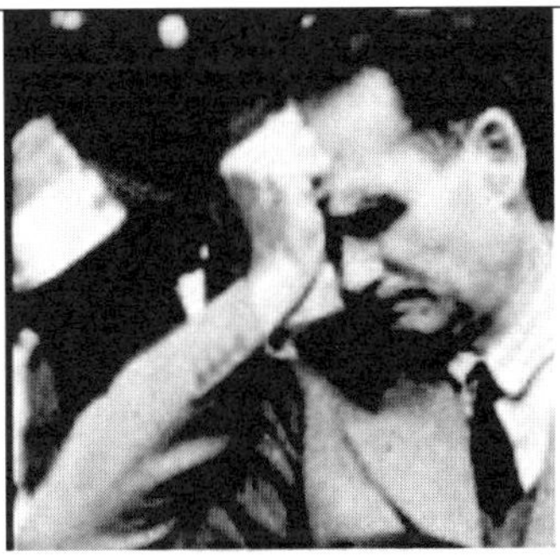

Rudolph Hess

Chapter 4

Rudolph and Hess Attorneys from Hell

It has to mean something when a Mayor named Rudolph will only hire Black men who share the same first name as himself. But when a mayor named Rudolph picks a corporation counsel named Hess, bells or perhaps air raid sirens should begin to alarm. I am certainly not the first person to speculate that something very Germanic must be going on up in Rudy's head, either consciously or unconsciously. Let us go to the symbols. Indeed, the name "Rudolph" does have Teutonic origins and memorializes the ancient Germanic people's celebration and veneration of the "wolf (wolph)." "Adolph," for instance, means "noble wolf" and "Rudolph" means "famous wolf." When Hitler's Deputy Fuehrer Rudolph Hess made his bizarre flight to Scotland, he initially denied his identity claiming to be someone called *Alfred Hayes*. The British Intelligence Officer interrogating Hess pointed out to him that Alfred was a corruption of the name of the first Saxon King called Alf The Red (Red Alf) and that in German this had become Rudolph. He also pointed out that Hayes was an Anglicization of the name Hess. The jig was, of course, up—although the famous face and Luftwaffe uniform had probably already betrayed General Hess.

I only recount this story in case one day when there is a war crimes trial in the Americas, a balding 5'9" pilot lands in Haiti claiming to be Alfred Julienne, the brothers and sisters will know who it is. It's the same guy who in 1982 claimed to see no political repression in Haiti. They should also know that if he is accompanied by a scholarly looking liar proclaiming to be Michel Hayes, it's really the mayor's attorney, so called corporation counsel, Michael Hess.

Slave Master Repetition Compulsion

If Rudy's actions against Haitian Refugees as Associate U.S. Attorney General back in the early 1980's represent a replay of the 19th century Fugitive Slave Act, then his actions in 2000 represent a replay of the Dred Scott decision. That's the case in which Supreme Court Justice Roger Taney said essentially that Black people have zero rights that whites are bound to respect. Hess, representing the mayor while testifying before the State Assembly On Codes, maintained that Patrick Dorismond's right to have his juvenile arrest records to remain sealed, ended with Dorismond's death. In other words, a Dead Black Man (identified with the N) word) has less than zero rights Rudolph and Hess are bound to respect. Rudolph and Hess cited as their rationale for releasing Dorismond's juvenile arrest record, the public's "right to know."

The same mayor and city law department that has offered countless frivolous defenses of the mayor's right to deny citizens their First Amendment rights and access to information via the freedom of information laws cites the publics' right to know. This is the same Michael Hess who represented the Federal Government versus The New York Times in a case better known as the Pentagon Papers case. This deceitfulness on the part of the mayor, is typical of persons with antisocial personality traits, persons commonly called sociopaths. Horse whipping would be too good! Since it might be illegal and would certainly be considered by some people unethical for a physician to recommend an Anthony Baez whipping or a Michael Stewart whipping for a prospective patient, I will say instead that the mayor and his partner could benefit from something on the order of a non-lethal Rodney King whipping but I would never call it that. No Rudolph and Hess needed harsh aversive behavioral modification which I will elaborate upon in my next book called - "Violence Therapy For The Criminally Sane."

Personal Injury Experts

I have a theory about what attracted Rudolph to Hess. It is not Hess' Phi Beta Kappa key, his having worked with Rudy in the U.S. Attorney's Office or his touted friendship with Rudy. No, it's something related to another of the mayor's quirks, Kennedy worship. Among Hess's credentials before becoming Rudy's first major appointment of his second mayoral term is the fact that he defended the Secret Service and Jacqueline Kennedy Onnasis in a case called Galella Vs The Secret Service and Onnasis. Ron Galella is the well known infamous paparazzi or aggressive celebrity photographer that hounded the Kennedy's in particular.

Rudy's obsession and worshipful fixation on the Kennedy's is well known. Other biographers have written of Rudy's having been moved to combat stance when someone spoke badly of the Kennedy's. Rudy, who attended Catholic schools such as Manhattan College and Bishop Loughlin High School (the same high school Patrick Dorismond attended) was so enamored with John Kennedy, the nation's first Catholic president that Rudy would sit with his college girlfriend, Kathy Livermore and say his own name aloud, "Rudolph William Louis Giuliani III, the first Italian-Catholic President of the United States."

According to Daily News writer Paul Schwartzman, they would even go to rallies for Robert Kennedy to pass out flyers. If that was Rudy's idea of a hot date, no wonder the relationship didn't last and no wonder Rudy had to turn within to his own family for a mate. It is also no wonder that Livermore is quoted as rating him as just an "ok kisser." Livermore's revelations regarding Rudy also revealed a little more of Rudy's antisocial (criminal) assaultive traits that his paranoid tendencies caused him to project onto Patrick Dorismond. Livermore told of how a jealous Rudy once punched a guy out for just saying something to her that he did not like.

The Daily News reported on April 9th about another fight where Rudy invited a smaller guy to a fight out in the park and beat him up apparently as his frat brothers watched. The same two fights with a Black college age young man would result in Rudy calling the frat a gang, and perhaps saying of the puncher, "he spent a good deal of his adult life punching people." "May the dead rest in peace" —that's me, the intrusive first person narrator not Rudy—he has yet to say anything that is minimally civil about a young man who shared the same religion, high school and interest in law enforcement as he.

A Wolf Howls At The Moon; The Moon Never Howls Back

Yet, Rudy could fawn and obsess over the Kennedy clan, that had as much in common with Rudy as the moon to a wolf howling tribute to it. John Kennedy was a rugged athletic war hero. Rudy dropped out of ROTC because of punctured eardrums he had as a child and avoided the war with a deferment obtained for working in the office of Judge Lloyd MacMahon. John was considered a handsome bachelor who dated the Euro-American standards of beauty even while in the White House. Yet he maintained an image as a family man, "handling his business" with next to nothing leaking to the press. John Kennedy was able to exploit this family image to the point that most Americans idolized even his wife and children, Caroline and John John. This was true to such an extent that John Kennedy Jr. was affectionately called, John John, to his dying day.

Rudy's relationship with his subordinate Christyne Lategano has been so public you have to wonder if it's real. Magazines have published feature stories about it. Rudy's apparent attempt to perhaps cultivate a Kennedy type family image by naming his daughter Caroline and allowing his son to cavort at Rudy's first mayoral election led to most citizens who witnessed the, let's say, slightly more energetic version of a would be John John, ready to call for Ritalin. Also, no newspaper ever had to have a "Jackie Watch." Unlike Donna, Rudy's wife, Jackie Kennedy was always with her husband, John. John Kennedy was personable and had a reputation, deserved or not, as an advocate for equal rights for all. A song about his brother mused that " I thought I saw Bobby over the hill with Abraham, Martin and John." The name Rudy will never be added to a remake of this song. John Kennedy's father was a wealthy Boston politico with a pack of children and a background as a successful Bootlegger. Rudy's father, Harold, ran a bar in Flatbush. He and Helen Giuliani never had another child except Rudy. Could this early isolation be the source of those socialization problems discerned by Daniel Moynihan when he noted that the Senate was no place for Rudy to learn to work with others, or get group therapy?

Imitation of Life

I could go on to make the point all the way down to the futility of Rudy's cross combing in seeming imitation of JFK and RFK's sweeping hairstyle. In that respect Rudy is not only "No Jack Kennedy," He's not even a Dan Quayle! Neither has Rudy been able to capture the abrasive crime fighter or Civil Rights image of RFK during his stints as Associate Attorney General and U.S. Attorney. The closest Rudy ever came to a civil rights reputation at the Justice Department was by attaining the reputation for incarcerating Haitian refugees and administering a racist immigration policy at the Immigration and Naturalization Service. Robert F. Kennedy was allegedly killed for his efforts against organized crime.

In contrast, Rudy had one of his assistants, Daniel Perlmutter steal a quarter of a million dollars worth of cocaine and money from his office. If we are to believe the story, Rudy never realized it until notified by the FBI. And for all of the crime fighter publicity Rudy was not the one who successfully prosecuted JohnGotti. Much of the publicity about John Gotti, by the way, was generated by a man named John Miller who found his way into the Giuliani administration as an assistant to ex-top cop, William Bratton. Perhaps ironically, Miller is also, according to a 1991 article by Verne Gay, the godson of the wife of legendary mobster, Frank Costello. Rudy's big break in politics came when he was mentored by Judge Lloyd MacMahon, who is the person who supposedly prosecuted Frank Costello. Think like a crime detective or a conspiracy theorist—But don't snitch.

No, Rudy's fixation and identification with the Kennedy Family, has nothing to do with any real similarities. Rather it has every thing to do with his narcissistic tendency to fanaticize about unlimited wealth and power (to pass) and his histrionic desire to be the center of attention and in the spotlight. It is my theory that Rudy's life skit involves the conscious or unconscious intention of trying to live out every character in the Kennedy Saga - everybody from John, Bobby and Teddy to the woman described by John prophetically as the late Miss Monroe. If Rudy's answer to any proposal (such as marriage) that *Christyne might make is: "We'll cross that bridge when we come to it,"* she'd better get in the wind. Remember Mary Jo Kopechne, another campaign worker who worked her way into *the* family.- but that and the Murdoch connection are stories for next time.

Quotation: *"Rotten teeth are strong against ripe bananas."*
Haitian proverb

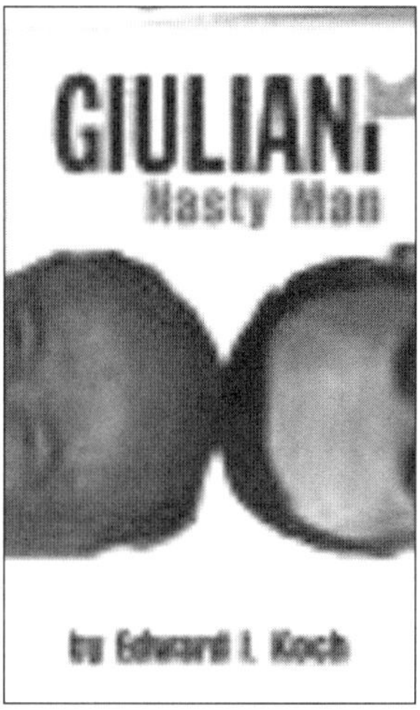

Chapter 5

Every Cigar Ain't A Cigar

Comedian, Red Fox once offered as a remedy for the common cold, the recipe of vodka and prune juice. Fox explained that it would not cure the cold - "but you'll damned sure think twice about sneezing." The moral of Fox's story is that every solution to a problem has potential fall out. So it is that the mayor has had to handle the analytical fallout of his solution to the problem of being perceived as self-righteous, thin-skinned and humorless. Rudy's solution was to participate in the so called "Inner Circle" charity show staged by a group of news people with past or present association with City Hall reporting.

At that show Rudy dressed up like Marilyn Monroe. He even imitated her famous rendition of the song "Happy Birthday" to John Kennedy. Clutching a big black cigar during all of this, Rudy, true to character even in this costume, demonstrated psychoanalytic preemption. That is, paranoid patients often try to anticipate the interpretation of their behavior or words by the analyst and utter either that anticipated interpretation or their defense against the interpretation before the analyst can say a word. For example, "I know you're going to say I'm projecting, but Black people really do loathe me." Giuliani in drag preempted interpretation of his phallic cigar with a quote from Freud. Said Giuliani, "Sometimes a cigar is just a cigar." But then again, most times for the psychoanalyst it is not, or Freud wouldn't have bothered to say that. Would he? And what about the blonde wig and dress?

Every Chocolate Malt Ain't A Chocolate Malt

If Giuliani would have us to believe that dressing in drag and smoking a big black cigar are anomalous events in his life, without meaning and not to be interpreted, then these events should not recur as the repeated props for the mayor's attempts at humor, but they do. The cross dressing found its way to the mayor again on "Saturday Night Live" some time later and the cigar figured prominently in an earlier prank the mayor pulled during his days at the Justice Department in the early 80's.

Newsday reported some time back that one of Rudy's coworkers claimed that on the morning after a night she, Rudy, and another coworker had gone out dancing, one of Rudy's friends told her that after they had parted for the evening, Rudy was arrested for soliciting a prostitute. The friend then led her to their mutual boss's office where she found in the boss's chair, not the boss, but Rudy, his big black cigar clinched between grinning teeth. So, analytic fallout not withstanding, Rudy's now habitual dressing in drag and clinching his teeth around a cigar got him through the annual Inner Circle charity event looking like a good sport. In so doing he lived up to the standard set a few years earlier when Ed Koch watched an actor representing himself sing a song called "I'm Koch" to the tune of Michael Jackson's hit, "I'm Bad." Lines from the song included the following: "My friends all lie/ My friends all cheat/ And as I sip on a chocolate malt /I tell New York, It's not my fault." If analysis were fair Rudy's foray into show business and cross dressing could only be interpreted in the context of the presumed mayoral normality of Koch.

Every Broken Clock Is Not A Broken Clock

But, Analysis is not necessarily fair and neither is an angry wife. Rudy's foray into show business required less of a sense of humor and less thick skin than his wife's most recent venture. It was announced last week that she will soon be starring in a play called the "Vagina Monologues" produced by a known political supporter of Rudy's rival Hillary Clinton. Give Rudy a "Broken Clock Award" if he thinks this has something to do with vengeance. As much as I hate to agree with anything Rudy says, even a broken clock is right twice a day.

Donna Hanover, Rudy's wife, long ago declared her sentiments to any awake observer, and I am not necessarily including the mayor among that group. In the wake of a rumored affair between her husband and his former communications director, Cristyne Lategano, Newsday reported that the relatively inexperienced Miss Lategano received a promotion that kicked her salary up to about $125,000. One of the reported perks was a new office in the basement with a private stairwell to Rudy's office. This was all reported in the context of Cristyne and the mayor in some folks' words, spending every waking minute together. There were even reports of them clothing shopping together on a Sunday.

Each of these news stories must have been like salt being poured into the wounds of Donna Hanover as she found herself publicly demoted from First Lady to Second Fiddle. Mrs. Donna Hanover Giuliani began expressing a preference to being called Donna Hanover. Rumors of Donna's squabbling with the mayor increased as their public appearances together diminished. These rumors began to explode when it was reported that the day after Rudy spent several hours visiting Cristyne in the hospital when she had suffered chest pains. Rudy emerged from home with a one inch cut on his forehead. Although Rudy throughout this scandal steadfastly denied any sex was going on, one pundit quipped that sex would make his strange attachment to this young staffer seem "less weird." Perhaps Daily News writer Sherryl Connely stated it best when she noted in an article that identified Cristyne and Rudy as a "Power Couple,""So united are they before the cameras, it's the First

Lady (Donna Hanover) who seems the other woman." Its safe to say the average woman would become angry about such rumors and such a relationship. Any suspicions on Rudy's part, that he's getting ready to get turned out by Donna's new career and social moves, have nothing to do with his paranoid streak. It is one of the ironies of paranoids that in the same way they are so suspicious when they should not be, they trust when they should not. Maybe he thought it was a coincidence when Donna appeared at a party hosted by Bette Midler in a skirt described as revealing while a friend dressed as a cop spoofed her husbands quality of life crimes crackdown by pretending to arrest her. He probably also thought it was a coincidence when she took a role in a movie about pornographer Larry Flint, who not only represents the opposite end of the spectrum from Republican Family values, but is known for a cheap shot he took at one of Rudy's icons, Jacqueline Kennedy Onnasis. Flint once published pictures of the nude Jackie captured without her knowledge, using a telescopic lens.

Every Monologue Ain't A Monologue

But no more exquisite revenge than her latest acting job could have been planned for a man with the control issues of a Rudolph Giuliani. The title alone "Vagina Monologues" could make him grow hair. The subjects dealt with in the play such as sexuality, orgasm, and lesbianism and the timing, right before the final election push, are "designer" wicked. Giuliani is "textbook" up tight and as the pressure of all this mounts he may exceed the limit of his ability to mentally defend.

He heavily relies on defenses such as denial, reaction formation and undoing as well as the paranoid defenses of projection and personalization discussed earlier. Reaction formation is the defense mechanism whereby a person handles an unwanted or undesirable impulse by resolving and expressing it as its opposite. The behavior pattern seen when someone uses this defense often seems exaggerated and inappropriate. If for instance an adulterer dealt with the issue of sex, he might go on a anti-porn crusade on some large street such as 42nd street.

Undoing is similar to this defense in that the person takes actions to negate or nullify past impulses or, undo the consequences that the person irrationally anticipates from a frightening obsessive thought or impulse. For example, if a person who led a police riot against a former Black mayor at City Hall that involved thousands of armed police rattling doors, banging on windows cursing out and shoving passers by, develops an obsessive concern for safety issues at City Hall to the point of building protective barricades and ignoring all court orders restricting him from doing so, a certain amount of undoing may be at play, as well as the more obvious defense of projection.

A person, who was characterized as a nerd at college, must constantly guard against that image reoccurring in his mind by making macho power moves such as permitting an airplane to buzz a crowd of a few thousand youth at a rally in Harlem. That could be perceived as undoing. In the instance of the first Million Youth March, held in July the mayor became fearful that the demonstrators would attempt to extend their rally a few moments past the allocated time, so, he permitted the police to charge the demonstrators in a full on frontal assault, Bay of Pigs style. He thereby insured that the city would have to deal with the aftermath of the demonstration, not for just a few moments, but legally, financially, medically, and politically for a few years. This tendency of missing the forest for the trees is typical for the rigid obsessive, self- righteous component of Giuliani's character structure.

Every Controller Ain't In Control

He is a Kennedy worshipper perpetually trapped in a replay of the Cuban Missile Crisis no matter how small the conflict, dispute or grievance. A simple union contract results in him temporarily firing all the city's Legal Aid Lawyers. The mayor combs his pathetic balding imitation of Kennedy's hair then stares down the Ruskies and prevents nuclear warheads and Cuban cigars from striking Long Island City. The mayor is undoing every irrational and obsessive fear that comes to his mind.

We have had the Harlem Blockade for a simple rally. and the City Hall Park and City Hall Steps Blockade for the prevention of evil press conferences. We have witnessed the New Year's Eve Times Square Blockade, the Yasir Arafat to dinner Blockade, the Taxi Drivers Blockade and the Vendors and Street Artists Blockade. These compulsive mini-repetitions of the original Cuban Blockade miss the forest for the trees just as the year 2000 Blockade of Cuba missed the forest for the trees. Cuban babies missing medication, baseball fans missing baseball, and cigar smokers missing the acknowledged premium of all cigars is missing the forest for the trees. This particular flaw in the character of Giuliani is the line of fissure in a rigid crystalline character structure with five sets of facets, the narcissistic, the obsessive, the paranoid, the antisocial and the histrionic faces of the same character. It is toward this obsessive, self righteous, moralizing , controlling, compulsive component that his wife, Donna's recent actions will have their greatest impact. Losing control of his own image as reflected in his wife's behavior is something that has seemed to unsettle if not undo him in the past.

Every Cousin Ain't A Cousin

Although the mayor got an annulment to his first marriage because he did not know he and his first wife were cousins, others, who ought to know, said he did know. For instance his cousin/ brother in law Richard Peruggi, was reported some years back in the Daily News to have said regarding the matter "Rudy lied." The bridesmaid, Pat Rufino, is reported to have said regarding Rudy and his cousin/ex-wife - They always knew they were second cousins." Regarding the "ignorance of sanguinity" excuse, Ms. Rufino said, "Rudy decided or someone decided that that was the out they needed." Rudy's Uncle Rudolph told Daily News writer Paul Schwartzman that he knew. Newsday reported that Rudy and Regina, his ex wife, used to play together at his grandmother's house on Long Island. Certainly, Rudy must have noticed that there had also been somewhere a sole woman that both Rudy's father Harold and Regina's Father Salvatore called Grandma. The point is that when Rudy faces shameful information related to his wife, he goes primitive. Denial is a primitive defense. Any contention on Rudy's part that he did not know his wife was his cousin is massive denial.

And yet there are subjects that can make Rudy go even more primitive than that. For instance, once Rudy was on, "Open Line," a talk show on Kiss Radio when a caller named William asked him if it was true that he hates Black people because his wife left him and lived with a Black Man. Rudy just stammered and answered some other question. Yet, there is good evidence that the caller William was not that far off base. Rudy may have indeed been traumatized by the reported relationship of Rudy's ex-wife/cousin to a very well respected Black man named James Hall. Mr. Hall was an educator who worked at York College in a department that among other things helped improve literacy among Black students. Ms. Peruggi also worked there and the two were close. They were close enough for her to come receive Mr. Hall's posthumous award inducting him into the Southern Queens Park Association Hall of Fame. They were close enough for my source, who visited their home, to say they lived together and for Newsday to describe Ms. Peruggi as Mr. Hall's "longtime companion."

Ordinarily in New York such a relationship would be considered a commonplace thing, but because of the Mayor's rigid character structure and his policies seemingly directed against all that for which Mr. Hall stood, it derives psychiatric importance. Again, the defense mechanism here seems to be his undoing. Mr. Giuliani has been outspoken against exactly the kind of programs at CUNY with which Mr. Hall had been involved. Moderates and militants alike have noted the excessive and obsessive nature of the Mayor's anti-Black policies.

Every Uncle Ain't An Uncle

Reporter Bob Herbert, a man not known as a militant defender of the Black race, summarized Giuliani's position on Blacks in CUNY as follows: "Who needs remedial classes when you can send students straight to jail?" When Giuliani did his Marilyn Monroe routine with his big black cigar in his mouth several of his top aides joined him. One who refused to put on a dress was Deputy Mayor Rudy Washington, a Black man. When the mayor was being prepared backstage for his act, Deputy Mayor Fran Reiter remarked that "Rudy has to go to a place he's never been before." Washington quipped (Where) "Harlem?" When Giuliani sweetened with $1.1 million dollars, an unendorsed proxy apology for Mayor Dinkins to the Hasidic community for Dinkins' handling of the riotous aftermath of the vehicular slaying of young Gavin Cato, Dinkins went right at Rudy's "wife problem." With a perfectly straight face Dinkins told reporters, " In the spirit of faith and hope of this Easter and Passover week, I invite Mayor Giuliani and his wife to my home to meet with my wife Joyce and me... I extend my hand in brotherhood. I ask him to take my hand."

Richard Parsons, a Black Republican, once owned the distinction of being a Black man described as a friend of Rudy's. Certainly, no Black man can receive that appellation anymore. Yet Parsons refused to be a token in Rudy's first administration. Rudy's first announcement of his top level appointees didn't even include the 2 Black Rudy's that would later find their way into his government. There were no Black folks, but only because for whatever reason, Parsons did not sham for Rudy. Nobody does that to Rudy, especially no Black person. Rudy eventually evened the score by siding with Rupert Murdoch in a dispute over cable access rights with Time Warner that by that time was retaining Parsons as an executive. In that situation Rudy the friend, reportedly did not even give Parsons as much as a New York Yankee Heads up.

Former Giuliani supporter Floyd Flake admitted that the mayor whom he characterized as "megalomaniac," approaching "paranoid schizophrenia" seemed to be a "little worse," when it came to Blacks. Reverend Calvin Butts a minister who bore the wrath of the Black community for publicly embracing the mayor has recently taken to calling his policies racist. The point of reviewing the stance of these Black men who at best could be described as moderates, is that Mayor Giuliani does not seem to get along with any Blacks on planet earth. His obstinate, controlling, self righteous, obsessive component of his personality would probably cause him to answer "No!" to police beating victim Rodney King's rhetorical question, "Can't we all get along ?"

Quotation: *"I Am sorry if anything I said made you feel bad; I am sorry it didn't kill you. "* ***Dr Yosef Ben Jochannan***

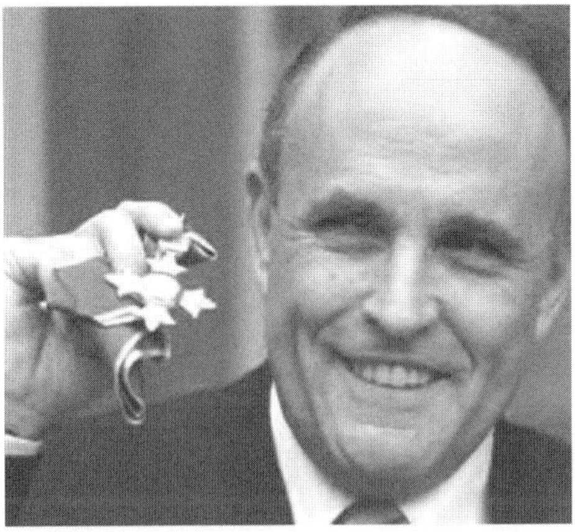

From Rudolph To Adolph?
"...the name "Rudolph" does have Teutonic origins and memorializes the ancient Germanic people's celebration and veneration of the "wolf (wolph)." "Adolph," for instance, means "noble wolf" and "Rudolph" means "famous wolf."

Chapter 6

Rudy's Mid Wife Crisis

It's been a milestone year for Rudolph Giuliani. He turned 55 years old. He's in the last term he can serve concurrently as mayor. The turn of the millennium has come and gone without the actualization of either theY2K disaster or terrorist destruction of New York City, both of which had consumed him to the point of building a $13 million dollar emergency command center (dubbed the bunker), building barricades around city hall and shutting down access to Times Square on New Year's eve. This is also the year he has had to finally put some distance between himself and Cristyne Lategano, a woman claimed by many to be his mistress. There has been nothing but changes.

Then last week, out of nowhere, less than one week after his 16th wedding anniversary, his wife announced she would be starring in a play called the "Vagina Monologues," produced by a supporter of his opponent in his upcoming senatorial race. In the script of Rudy's mind where he is the leading character, with a full head of hair and the body of a New York Yankee, the hero's back was up against the wall. What happened next, a press conference to announce his prostate cancer, will be for others wiser than myself to interpret, perhaps Mr. Tatum, (I only went to school for 28 years, and I cut a lot).

Kiss My Monologue

Is prostate cancer another wicked curve ball thrown at the hero, another tragedy, or the cavalry to the rescue, Deus Ex Machina, "God From A Machine," (translate this idiom as "a rabbit from a hat.") Literally, the public and perhaps Rudy, does not know which imposter this cancer might be, disaster or fortune. For catastrophe that cancer ordinarily might be, it has solved Giuliani's latest midlife problem which has been, of course, his wife problem. His wife, Donna Hanover, has announced that she has postponed indefinitely joining the cast of "The Vagina Monologues. And miracle of miracles, Donna Hanover (Giuliani again?) the woman who would not be seen with him in public a few months ago, also allowed him to kiss her in public and reportedly pledged to support him all she could. Even the spiraling decline Rudy had suffered in recent days in the polls has at least temporarily stopped, not reversed, but stopped its plummet. His political rival, Hillary Clinton, was even forced to say she joined the rest of the city in concern for the mayor's health. Mrs. Clinton is obviously a newcomer to town. Over two million people in New York are Black. And though the mixture of risk and rescue in Rudy's cancer announcement may have confused her, the white press to whom Rudy announced his illness and maybe even Rudy himself, it has not confused the Black community. If talk radio is any measure, there was little confusion about Rudy's illness and even less compassion and empathy.

Dry Hankies In The Black Community

As the week wore on, the questions Black radio hosts asked their audiences changed. Initially the question had been what do you think, or how do you feel about the mayor's cancer? As the hosts heard the answers, the questions on radio WLIB changed to, "Is it real?" or "Do you believe Giuliani really has cancer?" A surprisingly large number of callers to the station actually said they thought the mayor had made up the story. Some cited his calm demeanor. Indeed, the mayor demonstrated the classic stiff upper lip as he spoke to the cameras he had gathered together for his announcement. He said his cancer was treatable. He declined questions about his senate race and indicated he was going to focus first on the treatment options for his illness.

Perhaps even more surprising was the number of callers who indicated that they thought the mayor's illness was a punishment from God. On Monday of this week one caller reminded Mark Riley of the spiritual powers of people on the continent of Africa and in Haiti.

Many callers alluded to Rudy's behavior during the Amadou Diallo, and Patrick Dorismond tragedies. The words "What goes around comes around." were heard more than once. Indeed, it is a psychiatric observation that those patients who exhibit the least empathy for others often receive the least. During this season of milestone life catastrophes for Rudy, he was largely reaping the crop of his own long standing, narcissistic lack of empathy and obsessive need to stay in character as a macho lawman. Rudy's best friend reported to the Daily News writer Paul Schwartzman that he had only seen Rudy cry two times in his life, when his father, Harold, died in 1981 and when John Kennedy died in 1963.

Harold Wielded A Bat

If any two men are perhaps responsible from a psychiatric standpoint for modeling Rudy's public persona it is these two very different men, JFK and Harold. I have already mentioned the importance of the Cuban Missile Crisis to Rudy's psyche, but the role of his father as the progenitor of Rudy's tough guy image is probably even more critical. Ironically it was also the month of

April when Rudy's father, Harold, died of prostate cancer. But in his youth and middle age Harold was apparently quite the tough guy. He operated a bar in Flatbush and there are stories of how he would march into Kings County Hospital to confront people who owed a tab. It was even reported that he would smack a person around who didn't pay up. Certainly though in his bar it was known that he would use a bat on a customer, he felt, had gotten out of line. He reportedly preferred to issue a blow behind the legs. This preference would probably free him as a suspect for the busted eardrum Rudy acquired as a child - that is- if Rudy's Agency For Children Services had even existed back then.

However, I'm sure that more than one person has been arrested over in Flatbush during Rudy's administration for use or misuse of a bat, and that at least one youngster in this town has been removed from his parents care for as little as an unexplained busted eardrum. Paul Shwartzman also recounts a story of Rudy's being punished physically by his mom, Helen, on at least one occasion while as young as three years old. Combine these factors with a regimented Catholic School education from elementary school, where he was also smacked by nuns, through college and the kind of uptight pseudo-tough guy that might be produced was predictable. A wise therapist back then might have predicted that the chubby opera aficionado named Rudy, who was picked on for being a nerd and skipped his high school prom because he was so seriously considering the priesthood, would one day master overkill to the point of ordering police action to solve any problem from jaywalking to school tardiness.

However, something else altogether, of which biographers to date are unaware, must have gone into the development of this same man who will call a press conference for his own ailing prostate and is yet still so careful not to call the mom of an allegedly accidental police shooting to say something as simple as "mam, I'm sorry your dog, I mean your son was killed." No. Rudy's narcissistic lack of empathy must stem from something else they taught about in one of those classes I cut. It is as they say, at a "whole nother level." If Rudy had the slightest bit more humanity he could use this health challenge as an opportunity. He could say for instance, “I’m sorry everybody, I’ve been dealing with this thing for a while and it’s affected the way I behave. Mrs. Dorismond, Mrs. Diallo, Mrs, Rosario, Mrs. Baez, Officer Robinson ... can you forgive me?”

Are Dry Hankies Legal For Poor Folks

Don’t hold your breath. Rudy had to be ordered by the Federal government to even give applications for welfare, let alone assistance, or emergency Medicaid, to desperate people on the same day they applied. Black people who have faced catastrophe of the magnitude that forces them to endure a multiple visits to the welfare offices set up by Rudy and his “Work Will Set You Free,”(“Arbeit Macht Frei”) welfare chief, Jason Turner certainly couldn’t even be tempted to focus on Rudy’s prostate. Those forced to accept life in a distant homeless shelter in hostile Orange County (it should be called White County) at Camp LaGuardia would be equally unlikely to attend to the issue of Rudy’s ailing prostate. The Black father who witnessed Rudy’s police throw a concussion grenade into his home and yank his naked developmentally disabled, daughter out of the shower because they mistakenly suspected that drugs were in his apartment would very likely have to be psychotic to now weep for Rudy’s prostate. When the mayor has been so narcissistically non-empathic to the victims of his policies and even the alleged mishaps that arose from his policies, how could they be expected to concern themselves with the gland that produces his semen?

Indeed, it is in this dynamic between the Rudy that creates policies the courts have called illegal, that hurt people and the Rudy who fails to recognize the hurt and who even when recognizing it, fails to empathize with or feel it-it is there where the true interplay between narcissistic, obsessive and criminal self centeredness are revealed. The hidden crimes concealed by Rudy’s phony crime statistics are those committed against thousands of Black men and women who have been hurt and humiliated by the euphemistic phrase - stop and frisk. In Rudy’s lowest moment he will never empathize with the innocent Black youngster whose walkman radio has been thrown to the ground along with his dignity and self respect because one of Rudy's wild cowboys (spelled storm troopers when talking to Florida) felt like it or suspected something.

You could paint Rudy a thousand pictures or write a million stories about the grown Black men whose pants have been pulled down in public and he will never feel it. (Numerous reports of this on Staten Island emerged in the case of Ernest Sayon beaten to death by police for suspicion of drug possession.) . Lest it seem that I am waxing rhetorical, please recall that one police official got into trouble for having the modicum of decency to visit a woman in the hospital who required medical attention after police "by mistake" raided her apartment.

The Black Community Is Familiar With The Treatment Rudy May Face For His Cancer

Is it any wonder that many Black people cannot muster any sympathy for Rudy's cancer? Rudy's narcissism is itself a cancer and it has spread to the whole city. Any treatment of Rudy's mental condition must be drastic and must involve the entire city or Rudy can't be cured. More importantly, without such mass involvement the city can't be cured. What Rudy is facing now in terms of treatment of both his physical condition and his mental condition are nearly as catastrophic as his illness.

Basically there are four main types of treatments that have traditionally been offered for cancer of the prostate. All have potential side effects that no one, even a tough guy like Rudy, will want to face unless they absolutely have to. The first option is the surgical. If it were only benign prostatic hypertrophy Rudy would be a candidate for TUR or transurethral resection, something like a rotor rooter type operation with far less potential for side effects than the likely surgical approaches for cancer. No, for cancer any surgery will be more of the radical type reminiscent of the slashing cuts to welfare roles and budgets that Rudy made against the poor. A likely side effect to this is erectile dysfunction or impotence. A second treatment approach is radiation, either from an external source or from implanted radiation seeded directly into the prostate gland. This can of course impact negatively on the immune system or produce side effects similar to the surgical approach.

Many clinicians, however, believe that the impact of the radiation should ultimately be not too much worse on the entire body as the radiation of say a few of those X ray machines a person would face at the airport. So Giuliani should face such treatment with less concern than the average health conscious citizen who now cannot visit City hall without perhaps passing through the harmless X ray detectors Giuliani has now installed at City Hall Plaza. There are also some clinicians who offer chemotherapy with cytotoxic agents like cyclophosphamid and newer perhaps less toxic agents. Side effects of these chemicals can range from damage to the immune system to neuropathies (nerve damage.)

However, some of the newer agents in the hands of skilled clinicians are as safe as the harmless malathione Giuliani sprayed in the Black community last summer. Lastly, there is an older treatment, the hormonal approach. This approach involves the use of estrogens and some of the newer androgen blockers. These feminizing hormones have side effects that can include the acquisition of female secondary sexual characteristics such as gynecomastia (breast enlargement) similar to the sort that was discovered in 77 male Haitian detainees in December of 1981and again in 1982 in detainment camps such as Fort Allen run by the Immigration and Naturalization Service. Just to show you the power of free association, the Justice Department official in charge of the INS back then was Rudy Giuliani. Wasn't it?

You don't really suppose any of the callers to talk radio who said, "What goes around comes around," knew that , do you?

Quotation: When they want to kill a dog, they say it's crazy."
Haitian proverb

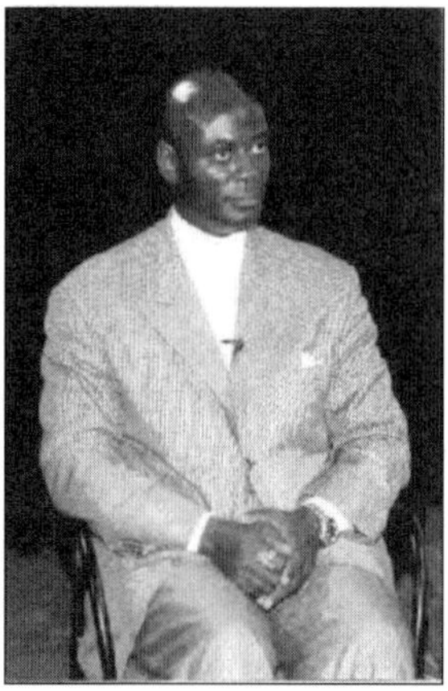

"There's a difference between Khallid Muhammad and me, and if you can't figure it out, you probably shouldn't be in the journalistic profession." Rudolph Giuliani - Newsday 10/19/98 .

Chapter 7

The Emperor Has No Sense

This week Reverend Al Sharpton took, what preachers might call, the high road regarding the personal life o Rudolph Giuliani. Sharpton refused to talk about Giuliani's reported girl friend, Judith Nathan,and refused to say, as many other Black New Yorkers have, that Rudolph Giuliani's cancer is a case of "what goes around comes around." Instead, Sharpton said simply, "I hope he survives, but I'm going to continue to fight him." Sharpton, of course, is considered by many to be the man who finally gave Rudy his come-uppance by organizing mass demonstrations of civil disobedience last year in response to the killing of Amadou Diallo.

However, it is another man who is not known for a role in those demonstrations who should get at least part of the credit for making them a success. That man is Khallid Muhammad. It was he who metaphorically proved that the Emperor Giuliani had no political, military or common sense. Muhammad, who was the leading figure among the organizers of the 1998 Million Youth March, had stood, again metaphorically, nose to nose with Giuliani and ultimately it was Giuliani who flinched by revealing a paranoid terror so monumental that he barricaded central Harlem, shut down subway service, mobilized the entire New York City police force and arsenal, including its air force for a demonstration of as few as 6000 unarmed mainly young Black folks. It was the criticism and ridicule that Giuliani received for this overkill that led to his tempered response at Sharpton's subsequent mass City Hall demonstrations.

In that respect Muhammad's role for Sharpton's success was similar to that described by venerated historian and ancestor, Professor John Henrik Clarke, of the Sikhs of the Northwest Province in India for Ghandi's success. The British knew that if they used violence against the non violent demonstrators of Ghandi, the people would turn to the Sikhs, who did not oppose armed self-defense. Sharpton was at the head of the line that columnist Jimmy Breslin had once predicted would form to be the second person to hit Giuliani once he was down. Well, Giuliani is down again and that line is once again forming. Like piranhas, New York's press corps, which has known of his relationship with a nurse named Judith Nathan for months, is now swirling around the couple, Donna Hanover and all connected to them, with biting questions everyday. When a Daily News Reporter asked police commissioner Safir if police were providing protection for Rudy's lady friend, Safir replied, "It's a nice day, isn't it." Wrong answer from the former law school attendee.

Waiting At The Double Crossroad

If Giuliani is sporting his new lady friend around with tax dollars, it's not just a nice day it's a perfect day - for piranhas. And sharp toothed piranhas are coming out of the woodwork. Former Representative Joe DioGuardi announced he was going to run (essentially as a spoiler) on the Conservative Party line for the Senate. Several top ranking State Republicans have also been quoted as mentioning a May 30th deadline for Rudy to decide once and for all if he is going to declare his already financed senatorial candidacy. The voices Rudy is hearing telling him that he's at a crossroads are not in his head. At least one is telling him he may be at a double cross roads. That is the voice of Liberal Party chief, Ray Harding , who has supported Giuliani in his two previous successful mayoral races. Yet, at this late date, Harding has not yet publicly committed to Giuliani and has recently met not only with Giuliani but also with his senatorial opponent, Hillary Clinton.

According to Amsterdam News, publisher Emeritus Wilbert Tatum, Harding is not the kind of person upon whose loyalty Giuliani should want to depend. Tatum wrote recently of Harding: "His religion is greed-any greed-for money, power or anything else that is negotiable. He is a dangerous man without a moral or scruple to his name. He would in all likelihood stoop to murder if could get down that low." If Tatum's assessment is correct, then Harding may go any way the wind blows, in light of Giuliani's recent behaviors. Giuliani's complex mix of character traits makes these recent behaviors quite difficult to assess. Are they sociopathic, manipulative, diversionary tactics to stop people from talking about Dorismond and Diallo? Are they paranoid pre-emptive strikes to ward off anticipated exposure of Lategano and other relationships? Or is this flaunting of his relationship the arrogant entitled behavior of the narcissist, the driven behavior of the love smitten obsessive or the attention seeking of the histrionic? Or are they just political suicide? I favor the last two formulations in my differential diagnosis.

Rudy's Hung By The Ties That Bind

Indeed, Giuliani's marriages and friendships- very good friendships have always seemed to have had the side benefit or perhaps main benefit of drawing attention to himself. It must have created quite a stir in 1968 when he married his cousin. Perhaps he had read somewhere of the blood relationship of President Franklin Delano Roosevelt and his wife Eleanor and thought this was a requirement for the office. One genealogist who studied the Kennedy's, John and Jacqueline, said that he concluded that nearly everyone was related to the Kennedys and the Bouviers (Jacqueline's family name) if he searched back far enough. Did a young impressionable Kennedy worshiper named Giuliani read something like this and think that marrying within the klan (pun intended) was the ticket to success? Or maybe young Rudolph was looking at what he thought was a potential connection to publicity.

Daily News writer Paul Schwartzman pointed out that Giuliani's first wife/cousin's father Salvatore was a broadcast executive. Her mother was a Rockette. If Rudy was looking for media exposure he may have married the wrong sister/cousin. Rita Marie Peruggi Mavromates his first wife's sister, (his sister-in-law/cousin) went on to also succeed as a media executive as producer with the Muppets outfit, Henson Productions, in the L.A., West Hollywood area (also called Safir-ville).

This Media/Kennedy thread weaves also through his marriage to Donna Hanover. Some confusion arose actually on the occasion of their first date, in that Giuliani's secretary seemed to think that Giuliani was meeting Donna for an interview and Donna thought they were meeting for a date. Hanover indeed confronted him on the secretary's mix-up. No one sympathizes with how hard it is for a businessman attorney like Rudy to keep his business straight. Donna also worked, as did briefly Jacqueline Bouvier (Kennedy), in the news business. Hanover's connection to media certainly did not hurt the career of a man who became known as the most publicized U.S. Attorney in New York's history. He has been accused of inventing the midday "Perp Walk" for accused Wall Street businessmen that he would parade publicly at the time of their arrest, allegedly in order to attract press attention to himself. It didn't matter to Rudy that sometimes these men would be found innocent. He would not let them, as had been the practice, surrender with their lawyers in private. This demonstrates that when he doesn't have Black folk's rights to violate, he's not above violating the rights of whites. The much publicized friendship/collegial relationship between Giuliani and his former Communications Director, Cristyne Lategano, also had its media value/ Kennedy connection. When Giuliani placed Lategano in an office under his connected by a private stairwell, speculation certainly abounded that he might be behaving in city hall as it has been written John Kennedy behaved in the White House. Lategano, if nothing else kept Giuliani in the news both intentionally and perhaps unintentionally.

Giuliani's most recent lady-"very good friend" shares the same first name as Kennedy's reputed mistress/ mob bag woman Judith Exner. Judith Nathan, R.N., was introduced to Giuliani reportedly by Elliot Cuker, Co-chair of the Mayor's Advisory Council for Film and Television, and owner of Cooper's classic Cars Cigars and Bar. The March 1999 internet version of nightclub.com magazine features a picture of a brunette woman sitting next to the mayor, who may or may not be Nurse Nathan. Cuker's face is next to theirs in the background, either sitting next to or leaning into one of the convertibles or convertible like tables at Cuker's Bar. Cuker has denied to the press that he has knowledge of Judith Nathan having ever frequented the club.

This notwithstanding, no one can deny that Giuliani's very good friendships with both Nathan and Cuker have kept him in the press. Cuker and Giuliani share what seems to border on a cigar fetish. They reportedly frequented so-called Cigar Bars. At Cuker's club humidors are rented at a cost of $1000.00 per year for patrons to store their favorite brands of cigars.

Everybody knows that Rudy is all man, but what psychiatrist, Dr. Frances Cress Welsing, has written about cigars in a paper called "The Symbolism of Smoking Objects" bears mentioning: "The habitual pattern of placing the symbolic phallus (penis) in the oral cavity is one example of symbolic compensation for sensed male genetic and genital inadequacy. ... acts of placing the penis in the rectum or in the oral cavity also achieve symbolically the results of internalizing and ingesting through a gastrointestinal tract opening, male substance... which parallels the inhalation of smoke and the swallowing of saliva when mouthing a cigar...."

Cuker is also, by the way, credited by the <u>Daily News</u> with being the friend who persuaded Rudy to dress in drag at the Inner Circle show a few years ago. It's a long fall for Rudy who stayed home from his high school prom because he was contemplating the priesthood and whose best friend Alan went on to become not only a priest, but also a monsignor. To say that Rudy has been acting "Cuky" for a man trying to become a senator is an understatement both psychiatrically and politically.

Question: When Did Giuliani Time Begin?

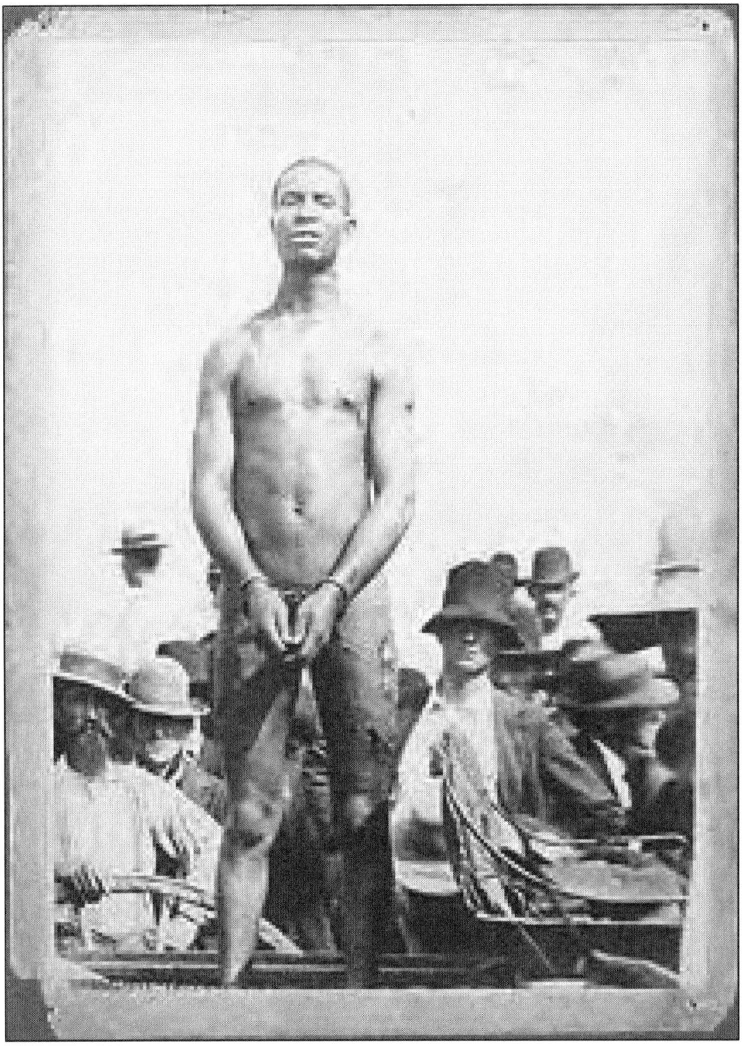

Quotation: "If you do not understand White Supremacy (Racism) – what it is, and how it works – everything else that you understand, will only confuse you." Neely Fuller

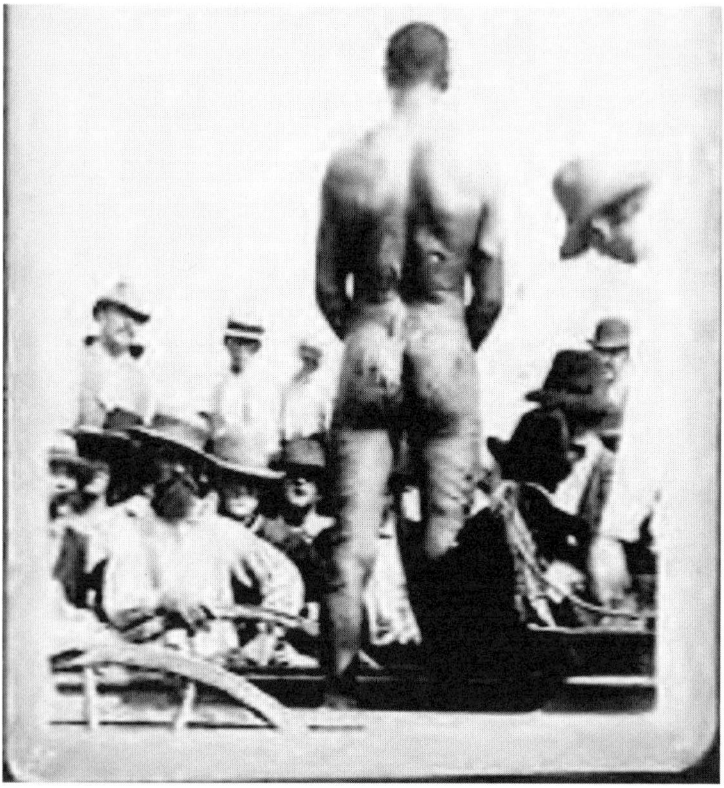

Slavery didn 't end in 1865 and Giuliani Time did not start in 1994.. In 1916 this man was tortured and forced to pose full frontal to the gawkers who then lynched him.

Chapter 8

The Other Tiny Bald Head With No Brain

Years ago, it was Mayor David Dinkins who noted that you can never say whether Giuliani has any political race absolutely won because, "You never know when he's going to shoot himself in the foot." The events of recent days with Rudy and Judy reveal that Dinkins had the absolutely right concept just the wrong appendage.

Until recently the only way Rudy could have lost the upcoming senatorial race to a woman he had dubbed a carpetbagger was by behaving exactly as he has. What married politician takes a very good girl friend to work with him without first going through the formality of labeling her a volunteer, an aide, a communications director or something? Then what politician jumps from the pulpit to the confession box then back to the pulpit again, screaming at reporters who are only asking about what he has already confessed to? For months the press had known about Giuliani's almost nightly dinners with Nathan, and had seen her hanging with his entourage so much that at least one aide reportedly thought she was a staff-member. Giuliani's refrain to the press since confessing to them that Nathan is his "very good friend" has been " leave civilians (Nathan) alone." He has even revealed that this edict is sanctioned by his apparent bible - The Godfather by Mario Puzzo," (Perhaps a chapter from St. Michael DeCorleone). Giuliani does not seem to know that as the chief civil servant he is a civilian and as the chief public servant he is public. Anybody he brings with him to public functions and secures with public funds is also public. Why should Nathan's privacy be respected anymore than Patrick Dorismond's? Why should her civilian status be respected any more than Amadou Diallo's or Malcolm Ferguson's? Giuliani, whose tradition as mayor has been undeclared martial law of the, "we own the night variety," now wants privacy. We have learned during his administration that "Military Justice is to Justice as Military Music is to Music." Just as we have been forced to learn not to expect Coltrane from a man whose heart beats to Souza, just as we have learned not to expect justice or mercy from a man whose soul resonates to Mein Kampf -- Giuliani must learn not to expect privacy and privilege from the long oppressed Black masses or the more general public. We remember how as a lawman with a badge Giuliani never prosecuted anyone for the violations of Eleanor Bumpurs, Yvonne Smallwood or Michael Stewart. These civilians' Civil-ian Rights were not important to him when he had a badge. Now as a civilian he boasts "I run the police Department," then bleats

"Leave the Civilians Alone." No very good friends of the Generalissamo (as he's been tagged in a book by a former staffer called "Sayings of Generalissamo Giuliani,") are civilians. Anybody who thinks they are is delusional. And indeed, of late Rudy, by his actions seems determined to make me revise my original assessment that he was not psychotic, and therefore not delusional.

Current Mental Status Report And Treatment

Yes, apparently bitten by either the love bug or his traditional parasite the shutterbug, Giuliani is talking strangely, acting strangely and feeling strangely (How's that for a brief mental status report?) but I am not revising my original assessment that he is essentially non-psychotic. I'm simply pointing out that even non-psychotic people with mainly characterlogical issues can disintegrate under pressure. When Hitler whose name "Adolph" as I told you means "Noble Wolf," began acting increasingly strange he committed suicide. When Rudolph Hess began acting strangely, he took a strange flight to Scotland, was imprisoned in England and eventually reportedly committed suicide. With this Rudolph (Giuliani) whose name means "Famous Wolf," political suicide via media seems to be his fate.

I had predicted in my first article in this series that you would hear an inevitable snap from the "bonkers bunker." This is it there will be no other. What treatment would I recommend for Generalissimo? - early retirement. During this early retirement Giuliani should repeat this mantra, I have never been the president, I am not the president, I will never be the president." Or alternately he can substitute any of the following words or phrases for the word president in the last sentence - New York Yankee, Jack Kennedy, Marilyn Monroe, the Supreme Court, or the Generalissimo. Giuliani does not have the nerve to take the noble route of an Adolph, nor should he. It's too easy given his crimes—and besides—we, the taxpayers, would have to pay for the cleanup. Giuliani's personal treatment is beyond the scope of any psychiatrist, no, an exorcist would be more appropriate. What needs treatment is the condition of the people whom Giuliani has hurt.

The Amadou Coalition on One Front, The Million Family March on Another Front and The Ballot on Election Day are all tools that can help our people—if not Giuliani. The Black Press has printed more of these chapters than I thought they would and for this, I thank the Creator for the Black Press. My apologies to those who feel I have gone into topics too low for discussion. Remember though as a propagandist, I do not score the touchdown, I try to tackle and throw blocks for the running backs, passers and receivers. Often I aim below the waist sometimes below the knees sometimes in the mud. I've been known to foul when the referees are not looking. I don't mind the flack at all if my people win the game.

Quotation: *Liberty is won with the edge of a machete.*

Antonio Maceo

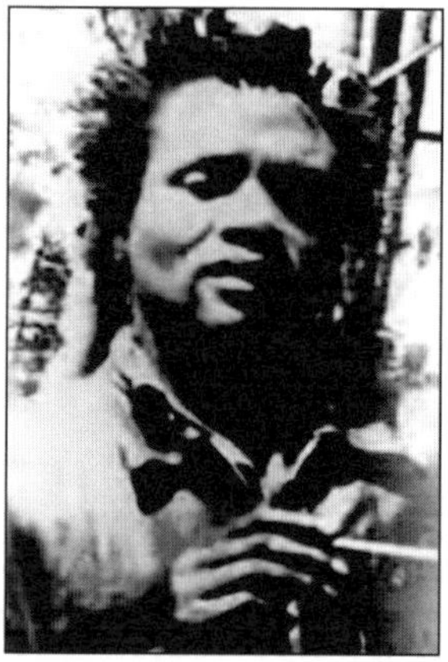

Dedan Kimathi of the Mau Mau

The same British government which honored Giuliani as a noble hung the "Kenyan Revolutionary Dedan Kimathi and ordered him to be thrown into a mass grave in 1957. The British government objected to and still objects to his reburial by the Kenyan people who honor him as a national hero.

Chapter 9

Giuliani and Spitzer: The Hijackers of Charity

So far, according to Attorney Alton Maddox, Attorney General Eliot Spitzer seems to have neglected his responsibility to prevent or stop a $10 million-dollar hijacking committed by Mayor Rudolph Giuliani. It has been reported widely that Prince Alwaleed bin Talal bin Abdul Aziz Alsaud of Saudi Arabia wrote a 10 million dollar check for the victims of the World Trade Center attack that has never reached any of the victims. It seems that the Mayor has waylaid the check and through his spokespersons announced that it would not be cashed simply because The

Prince had the temerity to suggest that U.S. Middle East policy was less than perfect. Alton Maddox notes that "Giuliani has no right to keep that check from the victims because it was addressed to charity." Maddox also asserted that, "Attorney General Eliot Spitzer has oversight over all charities in the state and has the responsibility to see that the mayor does not waylay that money."

Was The Bunker A Secondary Target

The Prince apparently had passed the check to the mayor at a ceremony commemorating the victims. It is only when it is recalled how imperfect the Mayor's own Middle East policy has been, that the significance of the Prince's generosity and the intemperance of the mayor's rebuke can be appreciated. Giuliani once refused to express condolences for the teenage son of a prominent Islamic leader killed by police and once personally barred Palestinian leader Yassir Arafat from a concert at Lincoln Center, despite the fact that Arafat had been invited. It should be noted that the suicide bomber pilots seemed to have been aware of the mayor's record in the selection of New York and the World Trade Center as one of their targets. The widely broadcast video of how the second plane seemed to precisely angle in on that tower suggests to some observers that Giuliani's nearby bunker was at least a secondary target. In fact the first building to fall after the two towers was the building housing the mayor's $22 million-dollar bunker called the Command Center. Two reports at the website of 1010 wins dated September 11th indicate that the mayor was actually trapped in his bunker for a significant period after the attack.

Is There Life After Suicide In Camelot?

Giuliani's hijacking of the check and his recent attempt to hijack his mayoralty past the State legislated term limits are clear indications that he has not been humbled by this near death experience in his bunker, his continuing bout with cancer, or any of the other catastrophic events in his life over the past year. His aborted senatorial bid, his very public divorce, his even more public alleged romance and unusual living arrangements have seemingly made him not the slightest bit less combative or rude. The events have also apparently made him no more financially cautious. At one point in the settlement hearings, Mrs. Donna Hanover Giuliani alleged that Giuliani's assets included the money left over from his senatorial bid. Using such funds personally is of, course, not permitted. Donna's seemingly, "off the cuff " allegation and perhaps veiled threat of exposure was not missed by many people other than Spitzer. Nevertheless even without Spitzer's intervention, the mayor for all intents and purposes was politically dead secondary to political suicide and mutual spousal character assassination.

However, as Camelot has reeled from September 11th''s brilliantly executed low-tech military terror, the mayor has seemed to experience one brief bright shining moment when it appeared that the reports of his political demise had been greatly exaggerated. Suddenly, people, the media mainly, were saying that maybe what the city needed during this crisis was some more of the mayor's iron grip. George Bush, who during his own campaign, distanced himself from Rudy's erratic behavior, even visited New York and later presented Giuliani to the Congress in Washington. People were saying Rudy could make a comeback and that Rudy had changed. It was totally possible that some of the people who said these things were serious. Others were, of course, simply being mischievous for the purpose of precipitating and witnessing one more pratfall by the mayor.

Mainly though, it seemed that the sympathy factor has been operating. People were simply being polite to this man who has long demonstrated less than optimal emotional regulation and has already acknowledged that he is gravely physically ill. The recent granting of knighthood to Rudolph Giuliani, who is to chivalry and nobility what Eliot Spitzer is to honesty and truth in lending was further evidence of just how finished Giuliani was and how much the sympathy factor is very much in play.

Spitzer's honesty to the Black community when he publicly promised to help attorney Alton Maddox regain his license will not be forgotten on Election Day 2002. Spitzer, Spitzer and Gambino, we specialize In 501C3. Neither honesty nor sympathy seems to be at play in Spitzer's willingness to look the other way at Giuliani's financial slight of hand. Spitzer, it seems cannot see wrongdoing in charity when the perpetrators are on Spitzer's side of the Middle East issue.

Neither Spitzer nor his former boss Manhattan District Attorney Robert Morganthau even answered a letter from CEMOTAP years ago, urging an investigation of the Anti-defamation League's practice of spying on Black political groups that was exposed by law enforcement officials investigating ADL's San Francisco branch. Spitzer, on the other hand, gets charity on his mind, and cannot seem to pass up investigating selected charities and even forming his own charities in the periods just before his political campaigns. Two years before his 1998 victory Mr. Spitzer and his wife Attorney Silda Wall Spitzer formed Children For Children Fund (CFC,) a charity which despite low contributions to the poor, has a board of directors that poured tens of thousands of dollars into Spitzer's campaign coffers. In the two years prior to his 1994 campaign, Spitzer's concerns had also turned to matters 501 © (3). He investigated the brothers Joseph and Thomas Gambino not long after it became public what heavy contributors they were to childrens charities. A children's bone marrow wing at Long Island Jewish Hospital is named for them. They, of course, are named after their father Carlo for whom the Gambino crime family was named. Spitzer negotiated a $12 million dollar fine, stay out of prison deal for the Gambino's in return for their promise to stay out of trucking in the Garment district where it was alleged that several pennies of every garment moved in the area had to go to the Gambinos. Spitzer, also at that time, formed the New York Chapter of Citizens For The Community Interest, a public interest group again with the initials "CFC" prominently in its title. CFC are also the initials of the "Combined Federal Campaign," the payroll deduction charity program for Federal workers.

I'll Watch The Money For You But Don't Watch Me

It is now 2001 Spitzer has investigated the financially solid Black run charity, Hale House ($10 million dollar endowment) and valuable real estate bordering Central park centering the real estate investments of Spitzer, his family and close associates. This investigation, of course, permitted Spitzer to appoint a Board of Directors. The Board of directors should of course have access to the charity's most valuable asset, in an election year, its contributor's list. Spitzer also has one day after FEMA, The Federal Emergency Management Agency, announced its intentions to create a body to coordinate and oversee the over $500 million dollars of charitable donations to the victims of the World Trade Center attack, announced without even notifying FEMA that he was going to do the same thing. Can the 2002 election be far off? Is Spitzer going to name this effort "Coordinators For Charity?" Spitzer is quoted as saying that he wants to prevent possible "mischief" with the funds. What about the mayors alleged mischief. What about Spitzer's own mischief - the $12 million dollars of campaign funds for his last two runs whose source he could never seem to remember.

Quotation: *It would have worked if not for the fire.*

Mayor W. Wilson Goode

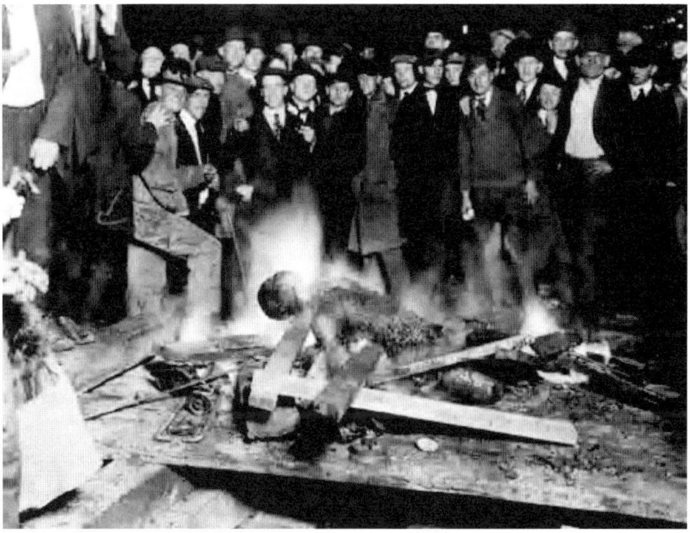

Chapter 10

Dum Dum and Dum Dumber

There is a story related to the origin of the word “Dum Dum.” It seems that Thompson submachine guns make the sound rat-tat-tat with ordinary bullets. However, if bullets are scored, hollowed out or in other ways altered to make them explode and expand on impact the sound of firing is “dum-dum-dum-dum.” It’s as if the inventors of these bullets knew who would one day be the police commissioner and mayor. Police Commissioner Howard Safir and Mayor Giuliani think the Diallo issue has been kept alive too long. Safir said in response to public officials being arrested, “It is now time to heal [not demonstrate].” A deputy police commissioner named John Timmoney once generously referred to Safer as “a lightweight.” Giuliani fired Timmoney for this insightful comment. If Safir should be called “Dum Dum,” what should the mayor be called?

The mayor says that the recent civil disobedience of Rev. Al Sharpton, former Mayor David Dinkins, Congressman Charles Rangel and two New York City Council members was a publicity stunt. For those who would dismiss the mayor's comments as asinine, be mindful of understatement. When Giuliani's police department came under fire for the infamous, so-called "friendly fire incident," where a white police officer, Peter Del Debbio shot a Black police officer, Desmond Robinson in the back four times, Giuliani engineered a press conference to make it appear Robinson said all had been forgiven. . Giuliani truly knows a publicity stunt when he sees one. Yet, his remarks are more than just the simple defensive projections of a master publicity stuntman. Giuliani's track record of sociopathy and media manipulation seem too extensive to permit Freud to excuse his hypocrisy. When Giuliani was the U.S. Attorney for the Southern District of New York, he captured more press than anyone in that position ever did. He deliberately prosecuted high profile Wall Street types, Democratic Party big wigs and flashy mobsters. It kept him in the press. He was both criticized and praised for his mastery of the art of riding the headlines. His career and political decisions all seemed designed to ensure a public presence. As mayor, Giuliani forced his own hand-picked Police Commissioner William Bratton, out of office for stealing too much of the glare of press flashbulbs. Even the personal relationships Giuliani has cultivated seemed to have some media-related objective. He had an early relationship (to be explained in a later publication) with the daughter of a broadcasting executive. His second wife was a news broadcaster. Chrystne Lategano, a woman with whom he currently has a close relationship and the person described by many as the co-mayor, collects over $120,000 per year for her ability to handle the press. To characterize as merely asinine, the remarks of a mayor with this history is certainly a mistake.

Consider the remarks Giuliani's police commissioner made four days ago regarding the cop detention of Nikkia Kelly, a teenage mother on her way to school. An undercover cop ,who should make all New Yorkers rest easier at night, stopped Nikkia to challenge her use of a student metro card. Since Nikkia was with a baby, the cop suspected she might be using her subway metro card to go somewhere other than school. Nikkia leaves her seven-month-old son, Kurtis, at the day care center at Julia Richmond High School, where she is admirably finishing her senior year. The cop made her late by detaining her when she asked to see his badge. Howard Safir called the arrest appropriate. That's asinine. Giuliani's words are not asinine: they are criminal because the loss of life is involved.

Giuliani and Safir took the opportunity of the Diallo mourning period to introduce the idea that if Diallo had been shot with hollow point bullets maybe his murderers would have had to shoot less. If Safir is Dum Dum, Giuliani is Dum Dumber. The outrageous act of policemen firing 41 bullets into an unarmed man has apparently piqued the consciences of nearly everyone but Rudolph Giuliani. The mayor has responded to the massive daily demonstrations of civil disobedience as though they are pesky over reactions to just one more insignificant dead citizen. Both Congressman Charles Rangel and Mayor David Dinkins could certainly get more publicity in a much easier fashion than getting arrested: Dinkins could get the front page of every newspaper in town simply by announcing that he was considering running for mayor again or by even announcing that Giuliani was no longer welcome to his house for dinner. Charles Rangel could share each of those front pages simply by hinting that he was going to run against Hillary Clinton in the Democratic primary for the U.S. Senate or by simply announcing that white corporations such as Rite Aid could no longer use the Harlem Empowerment Zone.

Sharpton, of course, doesn't even have to be defended. He needs more headlines, like Clinton needs more headlines. Sharpton, who is no stranger to Giuliani's criticism, was reportedly being maligned secretly by Giuliani via a conduit to Black politicians way back when Giuliani was in the Justice Department. Now Giuliani has a new more personal reason to criticize Sharpton. Sharpton is about the only New Yorker who can out-publicize Giuliani. What's worse for Giuliani is that Sharpton expresses no guilt or remorse for doing so.

When accused of being involved in a publicity stunt, Sharpton replied, "He is exactly right. Seven weeks after the fact, I am getting public officials to go to jail, to keep the issue alive." It is over the last seven weeks that Giuliani has lost over 20 percentage points of popularity. Now that's some publicity stunt! It is also the price that Safir and Giuliani are paying for being Dum Dum and Dum Dumber!

Quoatation: Can the devil fool a Muslim ? Not nowadays.
Master W. F. Muhammad

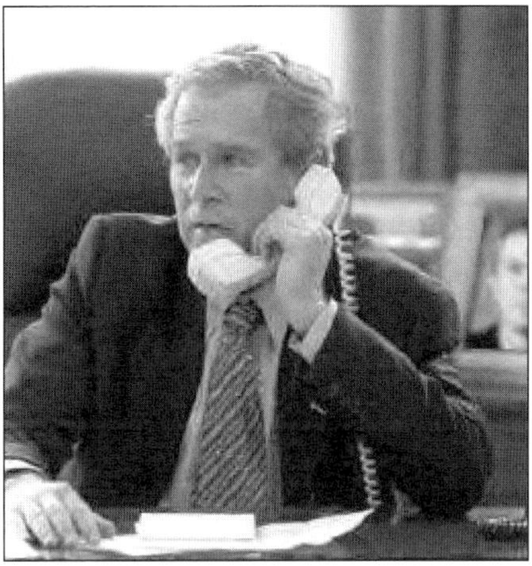

Chapter 11

The Zero of Ground Zero

Rudolph Giuliani after the terrorist attacks of September 11, 2001 looks like the same Rudy Giuliani, described in an earlier work, The Unauthorized Psychoanalysis of Rudolph Giuliani. He still demonstrates characteristics of the combined narcissistic, paranoid, obsessive, histrionic, sociopath, termed by The Diagnostic and Statistical Manual IV of the American Psychiatric Association, Personality Disorder Not Otherwise Specified. There is much evidence for anyone who will see, that Rudy the so-called *Hero of Ground Zero*, is really the *Zero of Ground Zero.* For instance, September 11th did not change Rudy's approach to racism.

The first thing Rudy did after the World Trade Center fell was to focus the city's attention on his traditional white super heroes --- cops, firemen and emergency workers. He had throughout his tenure done everything he could to make these already predominately white workforces "whiter." So when a catastrophe of this magnitude necessitated that he speak of the victims he found a way to only talk about whites. He pretended he was talking about heroes, but Giuliani's focus upon uniformed service workers was his device for avoiding mentioning Blacks even though that device required ignoring the Black Captain of the World Trade Centers Port Authority police, and a dozen of the firefighters who died at the scene. Ground Zero Rudy was the same old Rudy as he took photo-ops with whites and sound byte ops with whites and ignored the legions of Black dead buried at Ground Zero and the numerous Blacks, who by the mayor's definition of heroism, except for the color requirement, performed heroic deeds during the city's crisis.

All The Firemen And Policemen Were Not Heroes

Likewise, when the actions of the white policemen, firemen and emergency workers were less than heroic the Giuliani Administration positioned Black buzzwords as the perpetrators. Those few news leaks that emerged about the looting at Ground Zero focused on a couple of supposed corrections officers allegedly posing as police officers. However, the massive looting of apartments in the area and of the shops at Ground Zero could not have been done by one or two men. National Guard Captain Heintz, who spoke about the looting rampant at Ground Zero, pointed out that not all of the overwhelmingly white workforce and uniformed service workers at Ground Zero were such heroes. Heintz told the New York Times that the massive looting that was occurring probably involved policemen, firemen and other uniformed workers because it was virtually impossible for anyone else to get into the area. It should also be noted that Rudy took no blame for the reports that two possibly mob connected dumpsites were at one point getting the bulk of the scrap metal that was coming from the World Trade Center site. Stories about the corruption at Ground Zero never spread because of the information clamp devised and enforced by Giuliani.

Omerta At The Federal Crime Scene

Giuliani's long-standing assault on the first amendment and freedom of information act was continued after September 11th via a typically diabolical Giuliani distortion. He defined the area as a federal crime scene. He was, thereby able give the air of justifiability to his own quirky tendency to restrict information and access to information that many had previously termed paranoid. Likewise, Giuliani's very real obsession with crime continued at Ground Zero. It's a disguised but quite real obsession. Remember Giuliani grew up essentially in a mob family. His father was a convicted felon, a violent enforcer for a mob connected gambling operating out of a family pizza parlor. One might say, well that's his family and not him. However, if Mayor Dinkins background had been anything like Giuliani's, the press would have portrayed Dinkins as a probable mole for organized crime. If Dinkins' assistant had stolen a quarter million in cash and drugs from Dinkins' crime safe like Giuliani's assistant, a man named Perlmutter, stole from Giuliani's crime safe when Giuliani was a US attorney, Dinkins would have been called corrupt. If the scrap iron from Ground Zero had ended up in two Black owned dumpsites during Dinkins' administration Dinkins would have called a racist and corrupt mole. Yet the New York Press portrayed Giuliani as a crime fighter rather than a crime facilitator. Because of this, media brainwashing, some of Giuliani's hitherto worst critics have at worst merely damned him with faint praise saying, "Giuliani only did his job." The fact of the matter was that even at Ground Zero, he didn't even do his job.

Is Protecting Blacks From Racial Attacks A Part Of His Job?

There was a marked difference in the emphasis that Giuliani placed in his messages regarding the targeting of Muslims and Arabs for hate crimes and his warnings to perpetrators of fake terrorist pranks. Giuliani quoted Governor Pataki when talking about fake terror pranks. Giuliani spoke of really teaching a lesson to the first person that they caught. However, his admonitions against violence to other ethnic groups mentioned no punishments and were toothless perfunctory messages essentially to "be nice." There were no threats of teaching a lesson to anyone who targeted Arabs, Blacks or Muslims. Over the radio Giuliani's half hearted stammering admonitions against racial violence sounded like he was tongue tied and winking to the Klan, "You know I have to say this; the world is watching." This disparity in communication style regarding Black and white sides of the same issue was also demonstrated in all the mayor's communications regarding charity. The same man who required the largely Black poor of New York to appeal to the federal government to obtain the right to even receive applications for public assistance on the same day they were requested did everything but promise the victims of September 11th that they would get immediate assistance without hindrance as soon as they asked for it. He even established a special center for these victims and their families at a sequestered site along the Hudson River to facilitate the dignified and expeditious dispensation of aid to these victims.

The same mayor who once boasted that if things went the way he wanted, the poor would leave New York, showed that his callused attitude and lack of compassion are both largely reserved for those of darker hue. His statements and actions also exposed the fact that he had known all along how to dispense charity humanely, but simply had chosen not to do so. Giuliani's setting up special facilities for victims of September 11th by using city workers also represented a further siphoning to whites of resources from the underclass for whom those services had originally been developed.

Let Me Run The City For You Rookies Or At Least Let Me Handle Your Money For You

Selective compassion for heroes and whites notwithstanding, nothing could stop a person with Rudy's background from noticing the large amounts of cash that poured in around this disaster. Rudy clearly tried to do everything he could to remain in charge of it. He initially tried to extort an agreement from the mayoral candidates in this last election to permit him to run New York after his tenure as mayor expired. Then failing that, he via his supporters pushed to have Giuliani left in charge of the money through a privatization scheme for the charitable donations. Giuliani's ill thought out impulses as usual were not emphasized, scrutinized and ridiculed in the press had they been expressed by a Black. Nor were they acknowledged as errors by Giuliani.

Man Of The Year, No. Madman Of The Decade, Maybe

September 11th also brought no change to Giuliani's inability to admit a mistake. His multimillion-dollar bunker so-called emergency command center was about the first thing to crumble after the two towers. Twenty plus million dollars went down the tube for Giuliani's Boondoggle and not one life was saved because of its construction. Remember that it was Giuliani who asserted to his critics that one day the city would thank him for having built it.

Dinkins was harassed for purchasing an expensive headboard presumably for his wife and himself. Giuliani built a multimillion-dollar command center whose most popularized use was as a reported spot for he and his ex, Chrystine Lategano to spend one New Year's eve. This New Year's Eve, a televised kiss on the mouth of the new extra, Judith Nathan, puts to rest all the hopes of diehards who claimed that Giuliani's description of Miss Nathan as his very good friend was not intended to project the image that there was something going on between them. It was apparently very important for the mayor to publicly project the image of Miss Nathan as his romantic interest even as his wife and children exited Gracie Mansion. It was essentially his last act as Mayor of New York. The entire period after September 11th as well as this last mayoral moment does more to accentuate his past misdeeds than obliterate them. Man of the Year? No. Madman of the Decade? Maybe. *The zero of Ground Zero? Absolutely minus 273.16 degrees Celsius!*

Appendices

Each Appendix is a published article that relates to Rudolph Giuliani. Where possible, the date of the publication is provided. All of the following stories by Dr. McIntosh appeared in the Daily Challenge Newspaper. Many if not most also appeared in the CEMOTAP Drum. A few also appeared in the New York Amsterdam News.

Appendix 1

Daily Challenge
Thursday July 7, 1994

"Its not Dyson, its Giuliani, Stupid"

By James C. McIntosh

Deputy Mayor John Dyson recently came under fire for remarks many consider to be anti-Black. But according to many Black leaders in New York, it is Dyson's boss, Rudolph Giuliani, who "really hates Black people."

Words such as "white supremacist," "racist," and "right wing" recurred with uncanny frequency during separate interviews of activists conducted by the Daily Challenge. All but one activist polled used the word hatred.

Each of the activists cited their own evidence in supporting their opinion. Giuliani's policies regarding truants, his proposed policy to fingerprint welfare recipients, his use of disparaging terms to describe the homeless-"squeegee people"—and his frequent association with established bigots such as Bob Grant were among the most popular evidence cited of Giuliani's "hatred."

Activist Elombe Brath, chairman of the Patrice Lumumba Coalition, and a member of the December 12th Movement said that Giuliani's anti-Black policies are not a question of hatred. "He is a white supremacist trying to use such policies to his best advantage. He is a political opportunist," Brath told, the Daily Challenge.

Alluding to Giuliani's use of Bob Grant and Jay Diamond during his political campaigns, Brath called Giuliani "Bob Grant's puppet."

Activist C. Vernon Mason disagreed with the idea that simple political opportunism accounts for Giuliani's "anti-Black stance."

"Giuliani hates Black folks," said Mason. "He hates them because after his ex-wife (Marymount College president Regina Peruggi) left him, she married a Black man." Mason was referring to Peruggi's long term "common law" relationship with the now deceased James Hall, a former York College official.

"Giuliani is worse than Koch," continued Mason. "At least Koch had some 'House Negroes' in his administration. Giuliani has 'House white folks' and all Black folks- even the 'Negroes for Giuliani'- have to be in the field."

CEMOTAP's Betty Dopson, says that although "there's no question that Giuliani hates Black folks," she credits him with uniting New York's Black activists.

"We held a rally in support of Earl Caldwell and in opposition to the media cover-up of the white cop raping Black men in Queens. Groups from around the city, Marxists, Nationalists and others, with little else in common except their resistance to oppression and hatred, came together. Giuliani is a part of and symbolizes—the Hate Media Network to which Gary Byrd has referred: Giuliani is actually an announcer on WHateBC," Dopson noted. "His name comes up wherever you encounter racist media. It came up when the New York Post went bankrupt. And now that we've begun our boycott of the racist Daily News we find out that Giuliani. is propping up the News financially through proposed tax breaks and his successful attempt to let Daily News publisher Mart Zuckerman weasel out of a real estate bid he made for property in Columbus Circle."

CEMOTAP researcher Curtis Little blames Giullani's opportunism and hatred for his aid of racist media. "Some of it is Giuliani's hatred. ..But some of it is his vulnerability to media," said Little. "He is so vulnerable, I mean the wig, the marriage to his own cousin, the hysterical personality, the speech impediment. If he didn't suck up to the media, he'd be out of politics. "So it's personal and political," Little said.

Attorney Alton Maddox says he has "more personal evidence of Giuliani's hatred," Said Maddox: "A lot of people forget that Giuliani was the one a few years ago that came after me, Vernon (Mason) and (Al) Sharpton saying he had some incriminating tapes that a guy named 'Mclease' had made on us. It turned out not to be true. But I believe he was driven by hatred. Also remember that Giuliani never thought that any Black person's civil rights were violated while he was U.S. attorney: not Eleanor Bumpurs, not Yvonne Smallwood, not Michael Stewart - nobody."

Indeed, as Maddox points out, Giuliani does seem to have a blindness to civil rights violation. After John Dyson last week had a remark he made, published in The Bond Trader-in which he Implied that a bid by a Black firm for a city contract being considered by City Comptroller

Alan Hevesi was not to be taken seriously: "He doesn't know the difference between a bid and a watermelon," Dyson told the paper- Giuliani quickly accepted Dyson's explanation that tire remark was not intended to be racial.

Rev. Al Sharpton's remark on this is most to the point. "(Dyson's) remark was not made in the context of a discussion about citrus fruits. It was made in a discussion about a Black contractor," he said.
Giuliani, as has been his pattern, typically saw no violation and made remarks to the effect that he was standing by John Dyson. If Giuilani does not hate African people as many assert, he must have a very concrete and superficial understanding of racism. Dyson's clearly hateful slur is really not the most frightening aspect of the racism of Giuliani's administration, it simply represents it.
Giuliani's defense of the police "homicide" of Ernest Sayon and the explanation for why the homicide was not a murder is something that should be replayed on videotape for any who would become experts of doublespeak. As the anniversary of Crown Heights approaches, one must wonder if a boast made by John Dyson several months ago about two white guys having run New York for the last 200 years is truly reflective of the depth of Mayor Giuliani's insight. If he is ever to know the difference between a city and a watermelon, he should consider the words of his cousin and ex wife Regina Peruggi as she spoke at an event inducting a Black man, Dr. James Hall, Jr. Into Black America's Hall of Fame.

Said Peruggi: "One of the things (James Hall) taught us was the need for us to dignify people whomever they are." The "us" clearly was not her cousin and ex-husband, the mayor or his associate John Dyson.

Appendix 2

Daily Challenge
Tuesday, October 6, 1994

"Ward Blasts Giuliani"

By James C. McIntosh

FORMER Police Commissioner Benjamin Ward yesterday blasted undeclared mayoral candidate Rudolph **Giuliani**, "the leadership" of the PBA and PBA members associated with an unruly police mass demonstration held at City Hall two weeks ago. According to Ward, **Giuliani** "attempted to incite" rather than "pacify" the unruly demonstrators who stormed City Hall. Several demonstrators were publicly drinking alcohol and shouting racial taunts during the melee which was further escalated when a mob of plainclothes officers closed down the Brooklyn Bridge for over an hour. Ward also revealed that, already installed secret cameras in the vicinity of the disturbance have the capacity to monitor the square where the demonstration took place. He also said that for some reason these cameras were not turned on.

Ward indicated that the NYPD's Internal Affairs should have supplemented installed monitors with handheld cameras in the "Governor's Room," a room at City Hall that overlooks the courtyard. The city's former top cop called the behavior of the involved police officers "disgraceful" and called the entire demonstration a "political ploy. He said that the leaders of the demonstration knew that Mayor David Dinkins' measure already calling for a civilian review board had no chance of passing at the time of the demonstration. He cited the opposition of Archie Spigner, a Black city council member, to be the bill of proof of that. Asked what may have been the real motive behind the demonstration, Ward said that the ongoing police contract negotiations or perhaps police efforts to obtain Glock 9 mm pistols were the real object of the demonstration. . . .

Appendix 3

The Daily Challenge
Thursday June 16, 1993

"Keeping The Tapes On Hate Radio: Hate Gate"

By James C. McIntosh

GEORGE WILSON has monitored "hate radio programs" from a little room in New Jersey for over five years. Wilson says hate radio both enrages and disgusts him. And this is what motivates him to monitor the airwaves constantly. Wilson says he has gotten people fired for "broadcasting hate" and that he is currently out to "nail Bob Grant and Jay Diamond" (WABC talk show hosts).

At any given moment, George keeps six months worth of tapes of the most outrageous broadcasts imaginable. Ask for anything said by a "hate show host" and George can find it. He has a near genius IQ and a nearly photographic memory for numbers. Asked when did talk show host Bob Grant call Hillary Clinton "a bitch" on the radio? George, without hesitation, said it was "February 5, 1993 during the 6 to 7 o'clock hours." When did Jay Diamond call a caller "a Black Bitch?" George recalled the date as September 10, 1992 "at around 2:45 a.m."

If any doubt is expressed regarding, George's accuracy he will scramble to one of his boxes of tapes and pull out the exact cassette and cue it to the remark in question immediately. If he no longer has the tape, George can find an entry from among his exhaustive notes, complete with index and cross-references.

When did Grant "wish the president would die?" George thumbs through an index and corrects you. Grant said "it would be delicious if Clinton came up positive for H1V -not die."

"I can get the exact quote for you If you want."

Grant's "remarks are filed with 21 other entries under the category "Death Threats."

George is obviously a man who takes hate radio seriously. He is a man on a mission. Although George is white, one activist believes George Is "possessed by the ancestors." Others have labeled him "crazy" or more "obsessed than possessed."

George certainly has exhibited “obsession” In the past. He was, at one point, so obsessed with swimming that, according to him, he became the New Jersey high school state swimming champion in the early 70’s. And while on the subject of obsession, George plays a tape, he says, of Bob Grant threatening him over the airwaves while talking to a caller named John.

Says Grant: “He (George) is obsessed...He is a psychotic...he is in danger of getting himself in kinds of trouble he hasn’t dreamed of yet, because I do have certain connections, John. And if you’re listening, George, I may make use of those connections and get it over with.” George plays several other tapes with either Jay Diamond or Bob Grant, he says, speaking about him. On one tape Jay Diamond says Ominously, “I know your wife’s maiden name. I’m going to be In touch with you.” George says that shortly after this, a family member received a brochure for a “Gigante sponsored trip to Italy,” addressed to George and George’s wife in her maiden name. George pulls out the brochure and envelope as evidence. He also shows a picture of a dead fish and the envelope in which it was mailed to him. George then tells how Grant and Diamond later did an on-air skit about George being sent a dead fish. On several occasions police from New York or New Jersey have visited George or family members in an attempt to reach George. The dead fish incident was one such occasion and George presents a police property report from the incident. Another police visit occurred after someone allegedly threatened Jay Diamond’s brother, Seth over the phone. A third police visit was, says George, the result of simply complaining In the New Jersey Star Ledger about then talk show host Police officer Steve Rogers. Perhaps the most fascinating occasion of the police visits, says George, was immediately after someone used a very ingenious method of completely knocking Jay Diamond of the air on December 3, 1992. On that occasion Diamond had called into Bob Grant’s show, as he often does, doing one of his imitations of Mayor Dinkins talking about dildos.

In the middle of Diamond’s routine the emergency operator interrupts the call and In the course of announcing the emergency interruption says the first four numbers of Diamond’s home phone number 677-1. This forced the WABC station engineers to knock Diamond’s line off the air to prevent the audience from hearing the operator say 544. George, of course, has this entire Incident on tape. The police visited because they say the call originated~ from the home in which George resided at the time. George, who, as mentioned, has a near genius IQ, denies having made the call. George did, however, make an agreement with the police to never call Grant or Diamond at home in the future. George says that one of the Policemen - a "Detective Newham" - threatened to kick down George's door if he did.

George, who considers himself "a Born Again Christian," takes his promises as seriously as he does hate so he has not even called Grant or Diamond prior to that day, George's voice was as familiar to hate radio hosts and listeners, as it is unfamiliar to the rest of the world. They knew George, not only because of his frequent calls to their stations, but also because of the growing effective-ness of his campaign against hate radio. George was known for sending copies of his "hate tapes " to newspapers, politicians, the state attorney general, sponsors and even the president of the United States. George shows letters from various people who received his tapes, including a letter from the White House.

Although he is a born again Christian, George admits to an ability for deception In the Interest of justice. He demonstrates several of the numerous voices and accents he has mastered to get past the call screeners utilized at most of the hate show stations. He also reveals how he conducted many campaigns against the forces of hate, in the name of a one-man organization called Media Monitors. But, he had to abandon this tactic when a real organization called Media Monitors involved in marketing had their law firm notify him to "cease and desist" in using their trade name. George shows the letter he received from Media Monitors' law firm.

Eventually because of his work, George became one of the most hated people on hate radio. George says that in the spring of 1991 former WWDJ and WWTJ talk show host Steve Rogers gave out George's full name over the air waves adding: "Do you want me to give out your address too?" In December 1990 George says that Rogers had police come to his mother's home. In July 1991 Jay Diamond, according to George, gave out George's full name and hometown over the air.

In an off the air conversation, according to George, Diamond warned him that he could have George "legs broken" and that Bob Grant could give out the word for people to hurt him. Also off-the-air George says that Grant told him in April 1992: "Your fate is sealed. When you don't expect it, you'll be taken out of the picture"

George's real notoriety began 1990 after one of his first victories. He succeeded that year in getting Steve Rogers out of station WWTJ. And George's notoriety grew as he became a ~particular thorn in the side of Bob Grant. In January 1992, George used his tapes to get the National Jewish Fund to cancel Grant as emcee of one of their events.

In February of 1992 George got one of Grant's callers suspended from his job as a teacher at Neptune High School. The teacher, David Clark, had called Grant protesting the fact that he had been instructed to teach certain materials during Black History Month.
On the air, Clark maintained that, "In 200 years we went to the moon. After 2000 years, they (Africans) are still over there urinating in their drinking and bathing water." George taped the exchange between Grant and the caller, then registered his complaint with Neptune school officials.

In a letter George later wrote to the Asbury Park Express on March 9, 1992, George said: "I feel sorry for David Clark. His career has been interrupted while Grant and WABC go on with business as usual." George continued to try to stop Bob's business as usual.

In June 1992, again by sending tapes to officials, George got Suffolk County citizens to cancel their planned "Bob Grant Day."
In July 1992 George got the international Immigrant Parade to cancel Grant as their scheduled Grand Marshall. George has become Increasingly frustrated in his attempt to get the people responsible to do something about Grant and Diamond. He has sent tapes to WABC program director, John Mainelli, to the Capital Cities president of broadcasting and to 20 Of WABC's sponsors, mainly to no avail.

Most recently, George has taken to sending tapes to Black organizations and leaders. He has sent tapes also to the major Black media outlets, and is waiting to see the response that is generated. CEMOTAP as it was reported in the Daily Challenge of June 3, 1993 has mailed information from 14 statements contained on just one of George's tapes to the Federal Communications Commission and various elected officials. Most of the Black recipients of George's tape have had nothing but praise for his work.

When one CEMOTAP member was asked whether or not he thought George was possessed, said, "possessed, obsessed I don't care what! No one else has compiled the stuff like him."
George, in the meantime, although rebuked, unrecognized and living in fear- to paraphrase the commercial, keeps on taping and taping and taping…

Appendix 4

DAILY CHALLENGE
TUESDAY, JUNE 15, 1993

"A Bullet For Joey, New Jersey Media Monitor Fears For His Life"

By James C. McIntosh

GEORGE JOSEPH WILSON never knew several years ago when he began his one-man crusade against hate radio that he was beginning such a long and fearful journey. As reported in the Daily Challenge (July 10, 1993), Wilson's journey began when he simply started taping the hateful statements of radio talk show hosts and sending them to people he thought could help.

Although George has successfully gotten at least one host fired and one caller suspended, he has paid a terrible cost. He has endured repeated police visits to his home, a dead fish being mailed to his home and thinly veiled threats to himself and his family by callers and hate show hosts, some of which were actually broadcast over WABC radio.

George Wilson says that during a live off-the-air phone conversation, WABC talk host Jay Diamond actually threatened to have his legs broken. An ominous pasted-together note received by George in the mail yesterday, and displayed on today's front page is the most recent threat.

Wilson has also provided tapes of the on air comments of Jay Diamond and Bob Grant since June 10, 1993; tapes that he feels are related to this latest incident. On the tapes Diamond and Grant can be heard making repeated, often cryptic references to the names "George," "Joseph" and "Joey" (all names by which George is called, the latter of which he hates). There are also frequent references to the town of Westfield, New Jersey, George's home town, frequent references to the police and some of George's recent actions against hate radio callers.
On the tape of June 11, 1993 Bob Grant can be heard announcing in his best 'mobster impersonation' as he exposes his appreciation to the Westfield Police for providing him with "inside information which will be very valuable."

During the same program, Grant asks his traffic reporter Noland) several times to verify that his name is "not Joey" and not "George Joseph Noland." Grant then tells Noland: "The Westfield Police were everything you say they are, a great bunch of guys, a great bunch of guys." Noland responds, "That whole Police Department - wall to wall -Bob Grant Country."

Then as if to be sure George got his message, Grant asks: "And they don't like if Bob Grant is - uh - is being taken advantage of'?"
"No they don't," responds Noland. On June 10, after a harangue about people who "like to make trouble for other people and reveal things of a private nature," Diamond says the following: "Mike Kochopoli is going to be here later to talk about 'Jurassic Park' and maybe he will also review one of the great, great all-time motion pictures, 'A Bullet For Joey. No such movie, of course, was ever reviewed.

Through all these unfunny and dangerous antics, Grant and Diamond seem to enjoy the complete support of WABC management WABC Program Director, John Mainelli actually faxed a letter to both the Daily Challenge editor Dawad Philip and publisher, Thomas Watkins, issuing threats on Friday. Mainelli also bragged about how many more listeners WABC had than the Challenge had readers. Said Philip in response: "WABC is powerful - no doubt about it. But we have the truth and - more importantly - the tapes."

Appendix 5

THE DAILY CHALLENGE
THURSDAY, OCTOBER 14, 1993

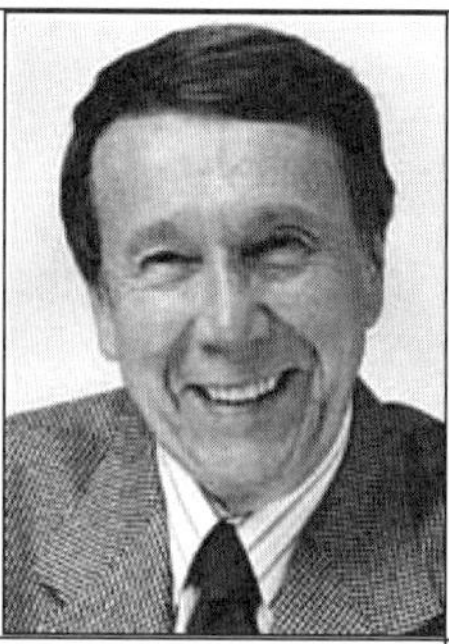	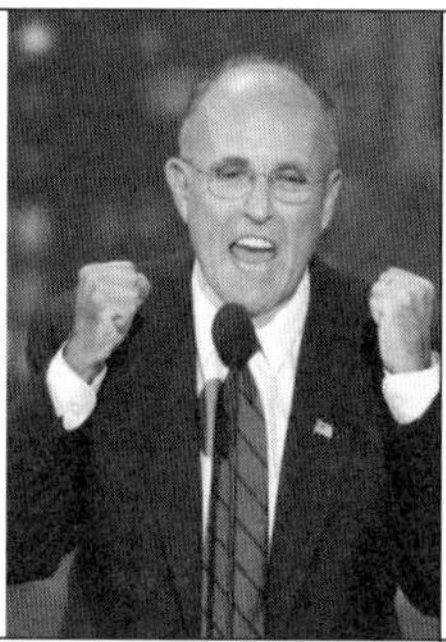	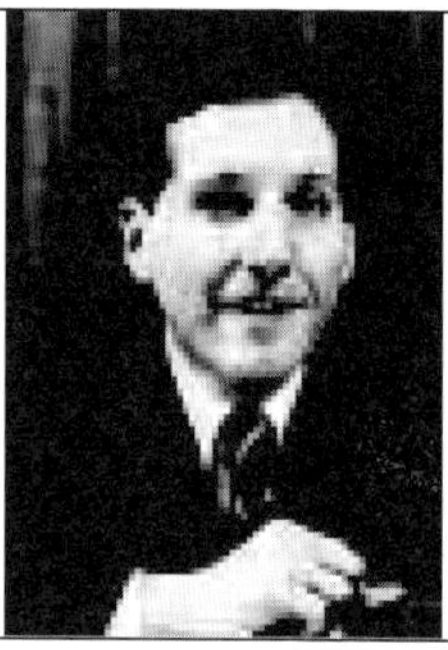
Bob Grant	**Rudolph Giuliani**	**Jay Diamond**

Grant"s A No Show At Giuliani Bash

Three things were missing from the Rudolph Giuliani pep rally held on Queens Boulevard in front of Ben's Diner on Queens Boulevard in Rego Park Tuesday night: a large crowd (only about 150 people showed), a jubilant atmosphere and the advertised guest speaker, WABC's "hate show host" Bob Grant. The rain could certainly be blamed for the absence of the first. But a grassroots Queens-based media watch group called CEMOTAP (Committee To Eliminate Media Offensive To African People) and the events they had sparked in the previous 24 hours, were the obvious cause for the absence of Grant and the presence of a tension that could be cut with a knife.

CEMOTAP Co-Chairwoman Betty Dopson - who had on the previous day (Oct.. 11, which she described as "Holocaust Day") brought 300 demonstrators to Grant's ABC studios to protest his well-known racial remarks - had announced that CEMOTAP would show up at the Giuliani rally because of Grant's scheduled appearance.

Dopson did show up with a band of less than 20 demonstrators who were able to visibly upset The Committee for Rudolph Giuliani, the event's organizers, and the evening's speakers.

Dopson's group braved threats from the angry crowd who shouted "Go Home, Go Home!" These chants were met by CEMOTAP's counter-chants of "Hate Radio, No Bob Grant, No Giuliani."

An especially tense moment came when an unidentified member of the management of Ben's Diner from the podium encouraged the crowd to physically force Dopson's group further back by crowding closer to the podium. The CEMOTAP demonstrators refused to move and police had to interpose themselves between both groups to avoid a confrontation.

The CEMOTAP demonstrators, who were noisy far beyond their numbers, became even noisier when Republican candidate for City Comptroller, Herman Badillo came to the podium. The group booed and screamed, "sellout" throughout his 20-minute attempt to be heard.

As the rally neared the end - and as the hour drew closer to the evening's planned highlight, Rudolph Giuliani's appearance police became fearful of violence should CEMOTAP demonstrators also prevent Giuliani from being heard. Two police sergeants, and eventually a police captain, tried to convince the demonstrators to voluntarily move away from the podium. Eventually the group was threatened with arrest. When the demonstrators still refused to move and insisted that they had done nothing disorderly or violent, the police set up wooden barriers and a double line of police to avert both violence and arrests.

A shaken Giuliani made his way to the podium to the snouts of "No Bob Grant, No Giuliani" from the CEMOTAP demonstrators . which continued throughout his less than five-minute speech.

Asked why she thought the event's "special speaker" Bob Grant had not arrived? Dopson said, "Grant is only fearless on the radio with his mouth. He is obviously a bully and a coward. He and his clone, Jay Diamond (WABC hate show host), target Black women, and other easy scapegoats.

"Also," Dopson continued, "Giuliani knows now after 300 angry African people - including Haitian activists and clergy - showed up at Grant's studio, that his (Giuliani's) free ride is over. He can't demand out of one side of his mouth that Mayor Dinkins denounce The Honorable Minister Louis Farrakhan, then out of the other side of his mouth laugh and act all buddy, buddy with racists like Grant and Diamond."

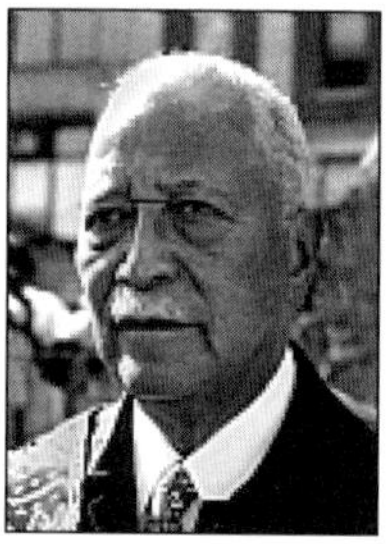

Appendix 6

The Daily Challenge
Thursday, October 26, 1995

"Guess Who's Coming To Dinner"

James C. McIntosh

On November 5 a dinner will be held in tribute to WABC "Hate Show" host Jay Diamond at the Hudson Theatre. Many of the characters one might expect to find at such a function will be there. The expected attendance of Roy Innis, Michael Meyers and Barry Farber will certainly not surprise anyone. However, one lady who says she will be there, Manhattan Borough President Ruth Messinger, will certainly be a surprise to a number of Black folks who have either helped her get elected in the past or who, even at this moment, are making preparations for her expected run for the office of Mayor of New York.

In an interview with the Daily Challenge on Monday, Messinger said she has "a record" of reaching out to various communities and is attending this function in that spirit. In a letter to Percy Sutton dated October 12, Messinger also stressed that same theme. "You may have heard," writes Messinger, "that I am identified as an honored guest at the upcoming Jewish Action Alliance event. I accepted that invitation as I accept others, in the spirit of engagement with a significant segment of my community"

Messinger wrote Percy Sutton not because the dinner will be a tribute to Jay Diamond, but because it will also be a fundraiser for the Jewish

Action Alliance, a group that this June boasted it was responsible for "every" demonstration against WLIB programming as of that date.

Messinger attempts to explain away her support of such a group in her letter to Sutton with the following: "I want to make sure you understand that in this particular case, among the issues I differ with the (Jewish Action) Alliance on are any attempts to challenge your license at WLIB."

Messinger said she was "unaware" that Diamond had done skits in which he spoke of teaching second graders about dildos so they would "not rupture their fragile little anus linings." She described Diamond having called a woman "a Black Bitch" over the airwaves as "reprehensible," but "free speech."

In her letter to Sutton, Ms. Messinger claimed: "I will always be consistently protective of free speech." Asked if she would cross a CEMOTAP picket line to attend the dinner. Messinger clarified the word "always" saying she would "cross that bridge" when she came to it. Said CEMOTAP Co-Chair Betty Dopson, when informed of Messinger's remarks,: "It's clear that Black people have to learn to build very different kinds of bridges with Messinger's community, the kind they can't cross or double cross.

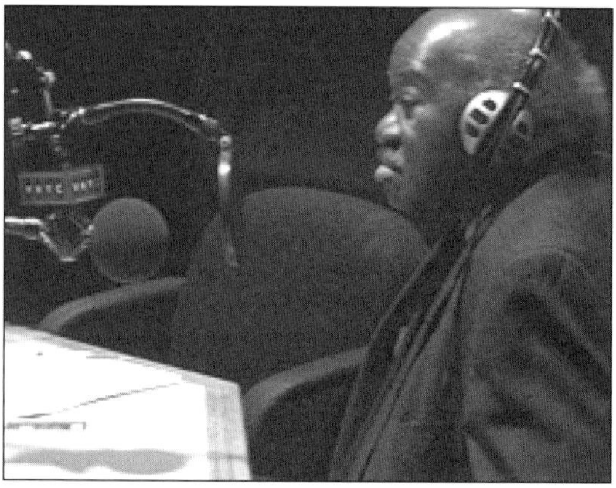

Appendix 7

The Daily Challenge
Thursday October 19, 1995

"Owens: Not Me At Diamond Affair !"

By James C. McIntosh

Susan Soneni, current press secretary for Brooklyn Congressman Major Owens, vehemently denied this week that Owens will be attending a black-tie affair scheduled for Nov. 5 at Hudson Theater. The event is being sponsored by The Jewish Action Network to honor hate radio host Jay Diamond and others. Soneni initially said she was not sure of the accuracy of an invitation she had just received from the Jewish Action Alliance that listed Owens as "Congressional Guest." After consulting with Owens, Smith said the congressman confirmed that he definitely will not be attending the affair and would like for the Daily Challenge to "make that clear" to the public. Diamond is known as a sharp-tongued antagonist of those he terms "the Black power left," a group broad enough to include writers as politically disparate as Les Payne and this writer. Diamond is best known for once calling a Black woman listener "a Black bitch" over the airwaves. White media monitor, George Wilson says that another part of the agenda of the Nov. 5 bash is "to raise a war chest for the Jewish Action Alliance to go after the operating license of Radio Station WLIB."

Appendix 8

The Daily Challenge

"Are Our Elected Officials Laughing At Radio Lynching?"

James C. McIntosh

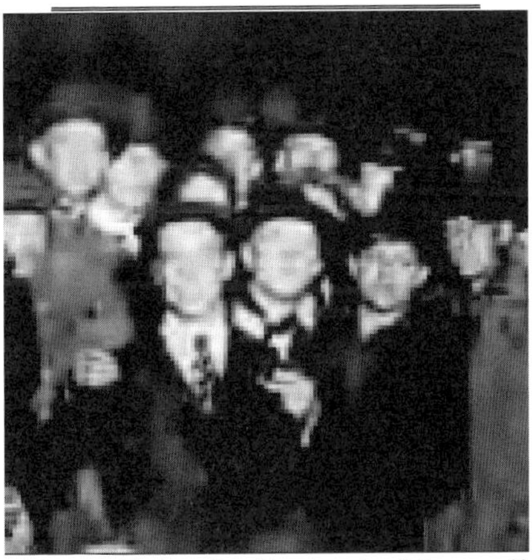

See Page 61 for the Context of the smiles.

The picture above at an actual lynching is taken from a CEMOTAP flyer called, "*Stop Radio Lynching*" CEMOTAP co-chair Betty Dopson held the flyer aloft as she explained the picture's relationship to a demonstration her organization is supporting. "If you look carefully in the background, you can see sadistic dunces grinning stupidly at their gruesome handiwork, the burning alive of a Black man "An examination of the picture revealed exactly what Dopson, said. "By honoring hate radio host Jay Diamond this Sunday," said Dopson "the Jewish Action Alliance is doing exactly what these men did. Jay Diamond is the radio host who called a Black woman a 'Black bitch' over the airwaves and who held mock executions or lynchings of Black leaders on his radio program."

Dopson also spoke about an incident in which Diamond broadcast a mock bombing of The Daily Challenge newspaper and the organization CEMOTAP, complete with the sounds of explosives.

"During one of his mock lynchings, I was mentioned by name. The sound of an explosion went off after it was announced that my body still had some sign of life, I was still moving," Dopson recalled. "To me, by supporting this event, Governor Pataki and Ruth Messinger are also doing exactly the same thing as the men in the background of this picture. "For me, it's personal," said Dopson, "not that hypocritical nonsense about free speech that Messinger is talking. Let someone talk about blowing her up and see how free she thinks that is.

"Professor James Blake of The Borough of Manhattan Community College seemed to be experiencing Sunday's demonstration both personally and politically. Blake, who was also the chief coordinator from Queens for the Million Man March, gave his reasons for supporting the demonstration. "We took a pledge at the march not to refer to any woman as a bitch," he said. "How can we allow our own elected officials, including a senator from Queens and the governor of the state, to pay tribute to a man who not only called a sister a that? We must register our protest now and at election time. bitch but a Black bitch. How could we call ourselves men if we did

Appendix 9

The Daily Challenge

"Marty Markowitz :"I Never Heard of Jay Diamond"

By James C. McIntosh

In an exclusive interview with the Daily Challenge, Brooklyn State Senator Marty Markowitz denied that he would be attending the Jewish Action Alliance Tribute to Hate Show host Jay Diamond and others at the Hudson Theatre on November 5. The issue was raised by activist Ed Barnes of CEMOTAP on Tuesday on radio station WWRL's Drive Time Dialogue. Markowitz admitted he may have lent his name to the affair (he could not remember), and admitted to having received an invitation to the affair but he was adamant about his lack of involvement in the event. "I never heard of Jay Diamond" said Markowitz at one point. "I have no role, I'm not even going ."Norman "Granddad" Reide, who is helping to organize a Black Men's March to protest the affair, said he is "angry" about "the nerve of a group honoring a man (Jay Diamond) who called a Black woman a Black bitch over the airwaves." Reide said he hopes that Black men from around the city will show up at 145 W. 44th St. at 6 p.m. on Sunday, Nov. 5. "The Sisters are excused from this one," said Reide. "It's time that we as Black men defend our sisters.

"CEMOTAP co-chair Betty Dopson said she was 'elated" at Reide's announcement. "One of Minister Farrakhan's instructions at the Million Man March was to support the Black press," said Dopson. "I'm glad the men are following through. This group that's sponsoring this tribute to Diamond has boasted that they have filed an FCC complaint against the city's number one Black radio station, WLIB. Stopping the Jewish Action Alliance in their fundraising effort is definitely supporting the Black press."

Appendix 10

The DAILY CHALLENGE WEEKEND EDITION, NOVEMBER 3-5, 1995

"The Bridge"

By James C. McIntosh

As early as October 12, Manhattan Borough President Ruth Messinger, in a letter to Percy Sutton, was explaining her surprising planned attendance of the Nov. 5 Jewish Action Alliance Dinner Tribute to hate show host Jay Diamond and others. .As late as one week ago, Messinger, in an exclusive Daily Challenge interview, also explained her intent to attend the same tribute. Asked if she would cross a CEMOTAP picket line to attend the affair, Messinger replied she would "cross that bridge" when she came "to it." Now, according to CEMOTAP Co-chair Betty Dopson, "Ruth has perhaps crossed that bridge a little before she came to it. "I have recovered a copy of a letter from Messinger to Beth Gilinsky backing out of the event. But even before I got the letter, my phone has been ringing off the hook," said Dopson."I called Eric Williams of WLIB news who told me that Messinger, in response to my criticism of her, claimed that she had not spoken to me in a year.

"She didn't have to talk to me about her intent to attend that tribute," Dopson stated. "She wrote her intention in a letter to Percy Sutton, which was shared with me by the Daily Challenge. There were news articles in both the Daily Challenge and the Jewish Forward documenting her intention." Now that she realizes that she's made a mistake, she should just admit it and not bring my name into it. "(But) with the heat that the Black men of CEMOTAP and other organizations are putting on elected officials associated with this tribute, I can understand such an evasive answer."
Dopson continued: "She joins a list of politicians who now say they will not be attending. Governor Christie Todd Whitman, Sen. Patrick Moynihan, Congressman Major Owens, State Senator Marty Markowitz and now her. We will be there—CEMOTAP will be there—on Sunday outside. And we will know which politicians try to sneak in and which try to sneak in representatives or written congratulatory

remarks. Now that Messinger realizes that—she has done the right thing, (for her) it's better late than never," Dopson remarked.

Appendix 11

The Daily Challenge

"Governor Christie Whitman: What Did She Know (About Hate Radio) And When Did She Know It? "

James C. McIntosh

New Jersey Gov. Christie Whitman admits that she is an Honorary Reception Chairman for a black-tie affair being held on Nov. 5, sponsored by The Jewish Action Alliance to honor "Hate Radio" host Jay Diamond and others. How ever, according to her spokesman, Ed Lake, a press staffer in her office, Whitman was "unaware" that Diamond had once called a woman a "Black bitch" over the airwaves. Whitman was also "unaware" that Diamond had once done a skit in which he joked about teaching "second graders" about dildos, so they would learn how to "not rupture their fragile little anus linings."

Whitman was "unaware" that Diamond held regularly scheduled "mock executions" of Black leaders on his radio program. Either Lake and Whitman do not read the Black press or they have read one too many of the maxims of Richard Nixon: "When in an embarrassing situation, stonewall."

Is it possible that Whitman could even claim not to know that Diamond had called her a "bitch" over the airwaves last October? This was not asked, but Lake did have the audacity to claim that Whitman was "unaware" that the group to which she had lent her name "for fundraising purposes," was raising the funds to assist the Jewish Action Alliance in their efforts to put Black radio station WLIB out of business.

CEMOTAP co-chair, Betty Dopson says that she is "dubious of Whitman's claims of ignorance, but will take the time to send her some material about Diamond and the so-called Jewish Action Alliance today."

"It's unfortunate, but quite possible," said Dopson, "that Whitman does not read the Black press and therefore has missed the dozens of stories about the excesses and racial slurs that are Diamond's trademarks. But she would only have to read the Jewish press to know that the Jewish Action Alliance is considered alarmist by even the larger extreme Jewish groups.

"Last June," Dopson continued, "they (JAA) wrote a letter to the Jewish Forward newspaper in which they criticized larger groups like the Anti-Defamation League of having no backbone. They bragged about how they had organized letter writing campaigns to WLIB's sponsors and had picketed outside the station. It has even been reported that Clayton Riley was let go from WLIB after he, quite appropriately, in my opinion, called their president 'Hitler's lovechild.'

"If I were to amend that appellation, I would only add the words 'spiritual mutant," Dopson said.

White "Hate Radio" monitor, George Wilson, who was responsible for sending tapes to Rev. Reginald Jackson and a group of ministers in New Jersey who were able to convince Gov. Whitman to sever ties to "Hate show" host Bob Grant, is willing to give Whitman the benefit of the doubt. "It's possible," said Wilson, "that she has not heard Diamond's worst stuff, but it's interesting that she has meticulously avoided being on Diamond's show for some reason.

"I would not call her a liar, though," said Wilson, "and I would e happy to help her learn the truth about these people." Wilson says he is hoping that Governor Whitman will follow the lead of Congressman Major Owens who informed the Daily Challenge of his intent to stay away from the November affair, even though he was listed as a "Congressional Guest" on the invitations.

Also, on October 1 9, Owens appeared on the airwaves of radio station WWRL and disavowed any connection to "hate host" Jay Diamond. Owens explained that one of his staff members had mistakenly sent his biography and photograph to JAA after seeing the names of so many other elected officials connected with the event. Owens went on to say that he and Jay Diamond "don't mix."

The following night, a miffed Jay Diamond implied that Owens was an anti-Semite and linked Owens' withdrawal from the affair honoring Diamond to "The Million Man March." According to Diamond's logic, it was funny how just four days after the Million Man March, Owens is refusing to attend "the Jewish dinner." Try as he might, Diamond seemed unable to rile up his audience at the specter of a new and dangerously anti-Semitic Major Owens. At one point, Diamond interrupted his tirade against Owens to complain that no one was calling in about the issue. Betty Dopson offered her opinion as to why. "People aren't going for the "okeydoke" any more. The portrayal of Black people as the planet's most dangerous anti-Semites is losing its punch. The fact is that most Black folks don't give a damn about what religion a white supremacist practices and—rightly or wrongly— most Black folks worship from a Bible which defines Jews are chosen people and identifies the son of their own God as a Jew. You can't get any more un-anti Semitic than that.

The Jewish Action Alliance is a fringe group that has been trying to break into the big time of alarmist fundraising for over a year now," Dopson continued. "People like Owens and Whitman will determine if they make it. What Whitman and the rest of these politicians had better understand is that Black people are in the position to determine if they make it. If she didn't know before that Diamond is a white supremacist and that JAA is raising funds to attack WLIB, well, what can we say. We're getting the information to her now. The question is not whether she knows, but if she knows that we know that she knows, and are going to hold her accountable for knowing."

Appendix 12

DAILY CHALLENGE
Tuesday, November 7, 1995

"Khallid Muhammad, CEMOTAP And The Boom Box Rebellion"

By James C. McIntosh

Over 300 Black demonstrators, including Rev. Timothy Mitchell, Norman "Granddad" Reide and Betty Dopson, laid siege to the Manhattan's Hudson Theatre Sunday night where the Jewish Action Alliance hosted a $150-a-plate dinner tribute to Hate Show Host Jay Diamond and others. Some demonstrators armed with boom box tape players accosted theater goers and tribute attendees with loud, looped tapes of Diamond saying his name, the radio station's call sign, WABC, and the following previously broadcast statement over and over: "You're a goddamned bitch liar, you're a son of a bitch of the worst stripe; and you know what? You're a Black bitch. You are a Goddamned bitch liar, you're a son of a bitch!

The main body of about 250 demonstrators stood directly across from the Hudson Theatre's main entrance and chanted the words "Diamond is a racist" repeatedly for several hours. One demonstrator wearing earplugs, drove slowly down the street with his car's tape-deck booming Diamond's cursing from the car's speakers. A squad of about 40 demonstrators posted themselves behind the theatre and another 25 posted themselves in the lobby of the adjacent hotel, which featured a side entrance into the Hudson Theatre.

Those tribute attendees who tried to enter by one of these more discreet portals found themselves surrounded and forced to listen to Diamond ranting "You're a Black bitch, You're a Black bitch" etc. Many expressed shock and disbelief. Others such as Golden and Michael Meyers, of the few handpicked Blacks attended the event, seemed to take the insults in stride. Nation of Islam Minister Khallid Muhammad coolly walked into the hotel to the cheers of the on looking demonstrators and asked for entrance into the tribute. Armed with an advertisement clipped from a newspaper that indicated entry could be secured by payment of $18O dollars at the door, Muhammad set the lobby into a frenzy of activity. With the most innocent of expression, Muhammad asked the hotel and theater security personnel who barred him entry "Why not? This says that entry at the door is $180 dollars and I have my $180," Muhammad declared. -

John Farrell, a white security officer, asked why Muhammad sought entry into the function. Again, almost innocently, Muhammad explained that "Mr. Diamond had spoken of him and he felt that perhaps Diamond might enjoy the opportunity" to speak to him in person, "eyeball to eyeball" This was apparently not the case, since Muhammad was never admitted and, according to demonstrator HilIy Saunders, "Diamond was scared to death.

"He came in about an hour early, so scared he that he didn't know what to do," Saunders noted.
Even so, Muhammad persisted insisting first on seeing the head of security, then, in a low courteous tone, demanded to speak to one of he tribute's organizers. Muhammad greeted many of the dignitaries such as Michael Meyers and James Golden with a handshake followed by a low volume interrogation. One white man, alarmed apparently at Muhammad "intense cordiality," said in a panic-stricken voice that he would not answer Muhammad's question until Muhammad, whose grip was apparently a little too firm and sincere, "unleashed" his hand. Later, a Black man who identified himself as the head of security, insisted there were no seats left inside the theatre. His announcement was met with jeers and laughter by demonstrators since so many of the featured "honored guests" had not shown up and whites who showed up continued to be admitted.

There should have been at least a few empty seats since none of the numerous invited elected officials were seen by anyone the Daily Challenge interviewed. A number of them had announced before hand that they would not be attending. Several, including Manhattan Borough Prescient Ruth Messinger, Congressmen Jerrod Nadler, Congressman Major Owens, State Senator Marty Markowitz, New Jersey, Christie Whitman and U.S. Sen. Patrick Moynahan, had announced previously that they were not coming—either directly or Indirectly because of the controversy surrounding Diamond's special recognition. Others such as ex mayor Edward Koch and U.S. Sen.

Alfonse D'Amato attributed their absence to the recent assassination of Prime Minister Rabin of Israel of the Black dignitaries who were to be honored, at least one was turned around after hearing the tape of Diamond. Rev. Betty Neal said she had no intention of going inside the tribute after hearing Diamond call someone "a Black bitch." However, when demonstrators perhaps half jokingly told her to go into the theater and bring out Beth Gilinsky, to face them, Neal took the request literally and actually brought Gilinsky back. Gilinsky, said by Manhattan Borough President Ruth Messinger to utilize an "up in you face" type of activism, apparently took Messinger accolade a little too seriously.

Backed by eight or nine males, Gilinsky crossed the streets toward the demonstrators. The demonstrators, who had already been loud, went ballistic, hooting and jeering her. Scores of them vaulted the police barricade and surrounded Gilinsky and her crew who opted to hastily retreat back into the theatre under police escort. In all, the demonstrators and police were restrained with the exception of one incident, seemingly engineered by the JAA and the police. After over an hour of refusing admission to Khallid Muhammad, word was suddenly sent to the hotel lobby that Muhammad could speak directly to Gilinsky regarding entry if he exited the hotel lobby (where hotel security was in charge) and came to the front entrance. Muhammad initially resisted this, but then walked to the front of the theatre with a squad of 15 demonstrators following him. As soon as Gilinsky came to the door, police rushed to the door. One of the policeman pushed a demonstrator. Someone pushed back and Muhammad had to step between the two groups to restore calmness. Around 8:15 p.m., the demonstrators disappeared as suddenly as they came, their mission accomplished. According to Betty Dopson, "We had won before we even came here. WhAteBC's dirty little secret is out and the Jewish Action Alliance has been exposed for what they really are. JAA is just Jay spelled a different way."

Appendix 13

The Daily Challenge
April 16, 1996

"The King of Hate Is Gone"

By James C. McIntosh,

Bob Grant's ranting is no more. He was called the "king of hate radio." Grant had insulted more Black people than the grand wizard of the Ku Klux Klan. But despite protests, letter writing campaigns and boycotts of his sponsors, Grant enjoyed a reputation as one of the most popular radio personalities in New York. A simple off-hand remark containing no profanity or racial slurs but issued against a dead man at the wrong time was Bob Grant's undoing.

On April 3 at around 4:58 p.m.. Grant said about the recently deceased U.S. Secretary of Commerce Ron Brown: "My hunch is he is the one survivor. I Just have that hunch. Maybe it's because, because at heart I'm, a pessimist" The expression of outrage at the tasteless remark issued from sources as varied as former governor Mario Cuomo to Rev. Al Sharpton. Only a few weeks earlier, fellow ABC host Attorney Allan Dershowitz had been fired for saying Grant was a racist. Certainly, Grant's position still seemed secured. But, a remark made about Ron Brown before his body was even cold touched a nerve that Grant's tasteless remarks about others had not. Grant had called the murdered 67-year-old grandmother Eleanor Bumpurs, "two ton Bumpurs." He had called Martin Luther King "a scumbag," Janet Reno "a dyke," Hillary Clinton "a bitch" and Gov. Mario Cuomo a sfacimm, (translations vary from scumbag to lowlife). So why did ABC decide to act now? According to fellow hate show host, Curtis Sliwa, Bob Grant was leaving the airwaves of WABC radio "by mutual agreement. No one believes this.

CEMOTAP Co-chair Betty Dopson whose group had planned a major demonstration in conjunction with Reverend Jesse Jackson and Reverend Al Sharpton today at 5pm at WABC radio, speculates that Grant "probably refused to apologize - The idea of apologizing to a

Black even a dead Black man—was just too much for the real sfacimm to endure. she said.

Appendix 14

Daily Challenge

"Hate Finds A Home at WOR 'White Only Radio'"

By James C. McIntosh

For a full week, a young white man named George Wilson had been able to relax. Two of his archenemies had seemed to be out of the picture. Former WABC Hate Show host Bob Grant, the man who had called Martin Luther King's widow "a skunk" had been fired for wishing the recently deceased and much-loved Secretary of Commerce Ron Brown dead. Jay Diamond, another WABC hate host, who had performed mock bombings of CEMOTAP and the Daily Challenge newspaper's office, had been on a suspicious leave of absence for several weeks, supposedly over a dispute for a better time slot for his graveyard shift hate show. George Wilson's dreams had briefly come true.

For George had for years obsessively dedicated himself to taping every hateful second of Bob Grant and Jay Diamond's radio programs. More importantly, George had mailed his tapes to anyone he had thought could help stop the hate. Wilson's tapes had found their way to literally hundreds of politicians, preachers and activists. George had lived to see governors of two states, assorted congresspersons and local assemblypersons denounce remarks by Grant and Diamond that George had taped. Nearly everyone admits that his tapes were essential in putting the nails in Grant's WABC coffin. George Wilson had endured death treats, slander, and police harassment and had even had a dead fish mailed to his home, but he never faltered.

However, on Saturday Wilson called CEMOTAP (Committee to Eliminate Media Offensive To African People) in a near panic: Bob Grant had been hired by WOR Radio. Eventually George's message reached CEMOTAP co-chair Betty Dopson. Dopson took the information in stride. "We are not going to panic." Dopson recalled: "On Saturday George called us frantically, 'White Only Radio hired Bob Grant, White Only Radio hired Bob Grant!' It took the brother

who answering the phone a few minutes to figure out exactly what he (Wilson) was saying," she said.
"WOR is 'White Only Radio' because they had never had a Black talk show host," Dopson explained. "What a more fitting home for Bob Grant's hate."

"But," said Dopson yesterday, "We are continuing just as we have in the past. If a powerful conglomerate like Disney/Capital cities couldn't stand the threat of a Black boycott, how could WOR and the Buckley Broadcasting Group stand it?"

Dopson said in the first hour of Grant's new WOR program monitored yesterday. "the sponsors were small home remodeling agencies for mortgage brokers. British Airways was the most vulnerable sponsor we've heard so far. But we are listening closely and by Saturday we should have a list of White Only Radio's most vulnerable sponsors.

Dopson says her group is hosting a program about hate radio this Saturday at 2 p.m. at 135-05 Rockaway Blvd., South Ozone Park, Queens. Minister Conrad Muhammad, activist Elombe Brath, and broadcaster Joe Bragg are confirmed speakers. George said his tapes are already hooked back up.

Appendix 15

Daily Challenge

"The Sickening Smell of Hate"

James C. McIntosh, M.D

Rev. Al Sharpton says that he is working to set up a meeting between leaders of the Asian and Black communities to put a stop to the bigotry spewing from radio station WOR hate show hosts Bob Grant and Jay Diamond. Diamond has been reportedly doing abbreviated parodies of the minstrel show "Black speech" he made infamous on radio station WABC during his mock executions of Black leaders. Then and now, Sharpton seems to be one of Diamond's favorite targets. But Sharpton's current focus is on a far more urgent issue. Sharpton and several other Black leaders say there is a clear connection between one of Grant's broadcast and actual racial violence that occurred against the Black and Asian communities of the Iselin-Menlo Park section of Woodbridge, N.J. in mid-December. "Clearly," said Sharpton, "one would have to be insane not to see that there might be a correlation between the remarks made by Bob Grant on his Dee. 11th broadcast and the subsequent Dec. 12th racial violence that occurred in Iselin, N.J." In that incident a store window was shattered by pellet gunfire, several businesses owned by East Indians and the home of one Black man was spray-painted with racist graffiti and swastikas.

Appendix 16

The Daily Challenge
Thursday May 2, 1996

"Inventing the numbers to invert the Color of City Government"

By James C. McIntosh

On Monday Mayor Rudolph Giuliani lied and said that there had been an overall increase in so-called "minority employment" in city government during his administration. Immediately Giuliani's claim was refuted. But, Giuliani is a man who can explain away anything. Instead of admitting his lie, he had his press secretary, Coleen Roche say, "He inverted his numbers." Oops! That's like saying Peter Del Debbio didn't shoot police officer Desmond Robinson in the back. Robinson's front was inverted around the bullets.

If that sounds too silly, remember that Giulinai's police department told a similar lie about the increase of bullets that have been fired since New York City policemen were issued the new 17 shot Glock 9mm pistols. A police study claimed a decrease in shots fired since their issuance but outside scrutiny revealed that police researchers left out hundreds of bullets fired during a big shootout in Queens where police in a classic overkill virtually machine gunned a restaurant The police have been shooting their new toys like bullets were going out of style. You can also bet that the increase in police brutality incidents are left out of any of the oft-quoted crime statistics issued by the Giuliani administration. Giuliani can of course explain that. These police assaults are not assaults because the police Civilian Review Board doesn't have the power to label assaults, assaults blah! blah! blah! etc."

But what does it prove except that Giuliani is the master of rationalization and half truths, and he will remain so as long as the New York press gives him a free ride. He is the man who saw no political repression in Haiti under the Duvalier regime only "economic" troubles.

Lest you think this was a simple case of again inverting the denominator, recognize that as reported in the Daily Challenge of October 21, 1993, Giuliani once appeared on a Bob Grant show where Grant called the Haitian refugees "savages" and urged mining the ocean around Haiti. And the mayor has returned to Grant's show again and again since then. Giuliani is not simply a lying political ally of Grant. He is much more dangerous than that. Giuliani has power! That makes him more like a Bob Grant with high impact. If Bob Grant is a "Dum Dum," Giuliani is a "Dum Dum bullet"

It was Giuliani's report when he worked for the Justice Department that provided the entire rationale for the denial of Haitian refugees the status of political refugees. It was Giuliani's lie that there was no political repression in Haiti that led to the establishment of a murderous Federal policy on Haitian refugees that was as effective as mining the oceans when one considers the number of Haitians who lost their lives as a result of that policy.

Make no mistake, Giuliani doesn't simply invert the numbers, sub-tract bullets and cast a blind eye to the victims of torture and repression. Giuliani invents the numbers, he hides the bullets and buries the victims. He is every bit the crypto fascist he was labeled by journalist Clayton Riley to be. But he doesn't lie because he's a crypto fascist. Giuliani lies because Giuliani is a liar.

He lies about simple personal and human frailties. When Giuliani's first marriage of over a decade to Regina Perruggi, his own cousin, was annulled, Giuliani didn't simply say 'I married the woman I loved, but it was a mistake.' Instead, he claimed ridiculously, that he didn't know she was his cousin. Did anyone ever ask him how he failed to notice at family reunions that they had the same aunts, uncles, cousins, nieces, nephews etc.? No! The press has never asked Giuliani these hard questions. They have never asked him if his hatred for Blacks is related, as Attorney C. Vernon Mason once postulated, to the fact that Peruggi eventually went on after her annulled marriage to Giuliani to live with a Black man named James Hall. Giuliani hasn't segregated New York City government. He has simply "inverted the color." He doesn't hate Blacks. There just aren't enough Black men named Rudy around to fill the jobs.

Appendix 17

DAILY CHALLENGE
THURSDAY, MAY 30, 1996

"Mayor finds out Blacks Can Be Rude-y Too"

By James McIntosh, M.D.

The mayor had come to WRKS talk radio program Open Line, perhaps expecting to be "Kissed" as the station's nickname promises. Instead, he ended up getting kicked to the curb by the largely Black audience.prepared with little speeches about drops in crime and the statistical insignificance of the decrease of Black faces in city government, Giuliani successfully talked right over the hosts of Open Line, Bob Slade, Michael Cottman and James Mtume. At one point, Giuliani actually shouted them down as they tried to interrupt one of his longer evasive answers. "Now, wait, now! It's my chance to speak," shouted Rudy.

An apparently fed up James Mtume then politely threw Giuliani to the wolves. "I wish I had two hours to deal with this, I want to get to something more we don't often have an opportunity to do, which is let our audiences speak directly to the mayor," said Mtume.The first caller pitched a softball question about education, to which Giuliani eagerly gave one of his stock answers about what he was doing for the children of New York. For some reason one of the hosts also tossed up a fat one to the mayor: "What is your opinion about Rudy Crew?" asked the host.

Like, what was Giuliani was going to say: "He's just like any other chubby Negro to me; I hate him." Of course not! Rudy extolled the virtues of Crew then got comfortable. That's when it became clear how badly hehad been set up. The next caller threw a mean bean ball. It was a hard, low fastball aimed directly at the lower torso. He began by asking Giuliani about his relationship with Bob Grant then from out of nowhere he lowered the boom with a follow-up: "Is the reason you have a deep-seated hatred against the Black community because after your first wife had left you and divorced you, she started a relationship with a Black man? And if that's true..." The hosts quickly— but not too quickly—interrupted.

For the next few questions, the mayor literally stumbled and stammered. At one point be even criticized "WLIB and WBBR" when he almost certainly meant to say WLIB and WWRL. The babbling of the mayor was sweet music to all Giuliani haters. One found oneself asking questions though, such as: Why didn't David Dinkins or the white newspapers ask Rudy questions like this and why didn't Rudy answer that question about the wife and the Black man?

Appendix 18

DAILY CHALLENGE

"Dinkins for Mayor Again Is No Joke"

By James C. McIntosh, M.D.

Former Mayor David Dinkins was sounding very much like a candidate for the upcoming mayoral race on his radio program "Dialogue with Dinkins," broadcast yesterday over WLIB. Dinkins' guest, Congressman Charles Rangel served as a straight man as the two politicians lambasted and ridiculed Mayor Rudolph Giuliani throughout the entire program. One of the biggest laughs came as they discussed Giuliani's threat/wish that he might prosecute one of District Attorney Robert Johnson's cases. Rangel, the straight man, gave Dinkins credit for "always" noting how the executive branch of government had to stay out of court matters. The two chuckled and expressed consternation at how Giuliani could ever consider such a thing. They literally stopped just short of calling Giuliani mentally unbalanced.

Giuliani and Police Commissioner Howard Safir had joined Daniels' parents, Curtis and Laura, in a heavily publicized vigil at their son's bedside. In the hospital, near Daniels' room, Giuliani embraced and kissed Mrs. Daniels before hugging other family members. Giuliani and Safir stood on either side of Mrs. Daniels. Rangel and Dinkins saved their biggest laugh for last as they discussed Giuliani praising the idea from a police memo that calls for frequent police sweeps of 125th Street as a way of engendering political support for the mayor. Although the memo announcing the plan was attributed to top police brass, Commissioner Safir later disavowed the memo as coming from an underling.

But not before Giuliani announced that the people of Harlem are against crime, too. The big joke is, of course, how could the mayor praise a police plan that the Police Commissioner disavows? Rangel and Dinkins worked it for all it was worth. All it needed was a laugh track," said Queens Million Man March coordinator James Blake. "It was all very very funny. But if the Black community laughs at Giuliani's first term serving as the Schools Chancellor, District Attorney, Police Commissioner all rolled into one, and then lets him have a second shot at it. The joke will be on us," said Blake.

Appendix 19

Daily Challenge
"Rudy Is Hard To Believe"

By James C. McIntosh

Rudolph Giuliani made only one true statement on WWRL's Drive Time Dialogue during the course of a half-hour interview yesterday. Giuliani was responding to a question from a listener about the double standard being employed by the N.Y.C. Human Right Commission as they investigated a claim by a reporter that she was discriminated against and denied entrance to a United African Movement meeting at the Slave Theater although the commission failed to investigate the mayor's refusal to admit PLO leader Yasir Arafat to a dinner to which 2000 other U.N. leaders and associates were invited. Giuliani, after initially pretending to know nothing about the United African Movement or the case finally said: "You're going to find it very hard to believe that I'm not directing what Curtis Sliwa does or (columnist) Minoo Southgate [does].

"I happen to know them, I happen to respect them. I don't direct what they do. They don't direct what I do. "And the Human Rights Commission, um, I'm not particularly involved in this investigation. They're doing it independently. And if you did discriminate and you did exclude people in a public place then they have a right to pursue you. If you didn't, then they are wrong and you're right."

See you all! The mayor can tell the truth! No, not the diversionary stuff about not being "particularly" involved in the investigation or the superfluous confession that he knows and respects Southgate and Sliwa. Remember that, coupled to the denial that he is directing them. The true statement—the one true statement—is the statement he made at the beginning." You're going to find it very hard to believe." That part is true! I do find it very hard to believe. I find it very, very hard to believe. But then again, you can't go by me. I'm a skeptic. I didn't believe the mayor's spiritual twin Mark Fuhrman either."

Appendix 20

The DAILY CHALLENGE
TUESDAY, JUNE 25, 1996

"Maddox To Rudy: "I'll Represent Myself"

By James C. McIntosh

Looking as though he could sing "Back In the Saddle Again," "Attorney-at-war" Alton Maddox yesterday left the New York City Human Rights Commission hearing beaming. He had just served notice to Administrative Law Judge Maldonado that he intended to defend himself and the United African Movement against charge of racial discrimination filed by columnist Minoo Southgate. Southgate says that she was denied entry into Brooklyn's Slave Theatre where, until recently, Maddox and the United African Movement rented meeting space.

Maddox maintains that even if Southgate had been excluded because of race it would not constitute discrimination because the occasion was a private meeting and therefore although the site of the meeting was a theatre, it was not being used as a theatre and was therefore not a public accommodation subject to regulation. Others have pointed out that in the hours before the meeting in question, Southgate and radio host Curtis Sliwa had threatened over the airwaves to come disrupt the Slave Theatre. Therefore, Southgate would have been barred, even if she was Black.

Seemingly with the laws solidly in his favor, Maddox has still maintained that he is prepared to accept whatever ruling the court makes with respect to the discrimination charge. "If they started ruling that private meetings have to be opened up to everyone, then I will be visiting some meetings of my own including the Trilateral Commission and the Council on Foreign Affairs to mention just a couple," Maddox stated wryly. "Either way, we can live with the decision."

Maddox was not, however, prepared to yield on the issue of self-representation at the hearing. "Requiring lawyers to represent people at civil hearings may support the full employment for lawyers, but it does not support the Democratic process," said Maddox. Members of Maddox's UAM organization and their supporters filled every seat in the hearing room. 1995. Diamond, who once called a woman a "Black bitch" over the airwaves, has also made threats in the past to march on the Slave Theatre.

Minoo Southgate, the complainant, actually had to sit at her counselor's table to get a seat. So Called Rights advocate Michael Meyers sat in someone else's seat but was eventually asked to stand to give a female supporter of Maddox the seat. "Mother Franklyn, an elderly woman member of the UAM, recounted Meyers predicament with a chuckle. "Brother Al (a serious looking UAM member) asked him (Meyers) to move to give the sister a seat and he got right up."

Meyers has often been associated with friends and associates of both Southgate and Mayor Rudy Giuliani such as "hate show" hosts Jay Diamond and Curtis Sliwa. Both Southgate and Mayor Rudy Giuliani and Meyers were scheduled speakers at The Jewish Action Alliance tribute to Diamond in November 1995. Diamond who once called a woman a "Black Bitch" over the airwaves, has also made threats in the past to march on the Slave Theatre. It is expected that if the proceedings eventually advance to trial, Sliwa, Diamond and Giuliani will all be called to testify. The mayor admitted last week over the airwaves of WWRL's Drive Time Dialogue that he knows and respects both Sliwa and Southgate. Giuliani has also offered his support of the right of the Civil Rights Commission to pursue Maddox and UAM if they excluded a person in a public place. Giuliani in November denied that he was "particularly involved" in this case. Giuliani will, however, according to Maddox, soon be "particularly involved.

"Giuliani will definitely be called to testify," said Maddox. The UAM chairman cited Giuliani's exclusion of Yasir Arafat from a U.N. dinner to which 2000 other leaders were invited as just one reason. Whatever the reason, supporters are looking forward to the prospect of "super defender" Alton Maddox facing in court the man who has represented himself as "super prosecutor" Rudolph Giuliani. Prof. James Blake, chairman of the Queens Million Man March Coordinating Council, is just one of the many who relishes the thought. Blake says his organization, along with CEMOTAP, is considering filing an Amicus brief in support of Maddox and UAM's position.

"If we can be forced to allow known provocateurs to enter our meetings," said Blake, "we are doomed. Because the mayor is an ex-prosecutor does not mean he can abolish the right of free association. He threatened to prosecute one of Robert Johnson's cases; I for one would pay admission to see Maddox face him in court and put him back in his rightful place - and believe me, its not in the mayor's office."

Today, at the hearing Maddox was in classic form as Judge Maldonado sought to set a suitable date for the next court date. When she [Maldonado] initially suggested the Friday after a holiday in late November, Maddox objected that the date was too soon after "Misgiving Day." The court erupted in laughter and a stony faced Maldonado set the date and place of the next hearing at December 3, 1996 at 9:30 am. at 40 Rector Street.

Appendix 21

The Daily Challenge

"Bob Grants Happy Birthday To Martin Luther King"

By James C. McIntosh

Bob Grant just doesn't get it. Kicked off of WABC last year for racist and insensitive remarks wishing death on Secretary of Commerce Ron Brown—literally moments after the fatal airplane crash that killed Brown—Grant has shown he is still a master of timing. Yesterday, as he has in the past, Grant used Martin Luther King's birthday for some of his special insults. While interviewing Bell Curve author Charles Murray, yesterday Grant asked innocently, "Why is it such a sin and a crime to acknowledge the findings of people like Gregor Mendel?" Mendel is the monk credited with outlining some of the fundamentals of simple genetics. The Bell Curve is the much-criticized book that purports to prove the genetically inferior intelligence of Black people.

Of course, the comment is mild in comparison to vintage Grant. Grant once called Martin Luther King , "That scumbag. Marty." However, after making' the remarks on Martin, Grant is still unrepentant for his verbal attacks on Black people in general, and Martin Luther King in particular. One of King's "Northern Lieutenants, Bill Morton, chairman of the Woodbridge New Jersey Human Rights Commission, and who 33 years ago was the central New Jersey coordinator for King's 1963 March on Washington, is fed up with Grant's racist comments. Morton says that racist utterances have led to racial violence in the past and that remarks Grant made about the Iselin section of Woodbridge, New Jersey last month led to specific acts of violence against one Black and three East Indians, Morton said that he has "picketed to have Grant removed from the air" in the past and accused Grant of "continuously inciting people."

To demonstrate Grant's effect on the Woodbridge violence, Morton offered the example he's seen of parents making racial remarks about Blacks in front of their children and then acting surprised when the children go out and trash a Black neighbor's property the next day. Morton, who is also the past president of the Perth Amboy branch of the NAACP believes this is what happened last month when Grant complained about the East Indians in Iselin.

On December 12, Grant whined about "the sickening smell of curry" in Iselin—as he has done on many times in the past. However, this time a few hours after Grant's broadcast, someone shattered a store window with pellet gun-fire and painted swastikas and racial epithets on businesses owned by East Indian and one Black home in the exact Iselin area of Woodbridge. CEMOTAP Co-chair Betty Dopson says Grant "has taken; his same racist act from WABC to WOR— White Only Radio"

"In 1993, while talking about the Iselin section of Woodbridge, Grant imitated an East Indian voice and asked: 'Does anybody here want to speak Hindu? I thought I saw an Elephant with Sabu." In 1995, on Martin Luther King's birthday, he commiserated with Neo-Nazi Tom Metzger about the court's temporarily blocking of anti-Mexican-Immigrant Proposition 187," Dopson continued, "He once called Iselin 'The Black Hole of Calcutta.' Now he airs The Bell Curve man and cheerleads some other Neo-Nazis into shooting into peoples' windows and painting swastikas; it's the same act, new station, same act!" Ironically, Metzger, the Neo-Nazi mentioned by Dopson, ended up losing his home when his Nazis were sued by Morris Dees, a lawyer from the Southern Poverty Law Center. But that only happened after an Ethiopian national was killed in Oregon following Metzger's remarks.

Is that what WOR is waiting for? WOR has made one cosmetic change after years of being White Only Radio: they have hired Luther Gatling, "The Credit Doctor." Gatling tried to remain strong and initially refused to go there as a matter principle over the Bob Grant issue, But, eventually, something lured him there. In case anyone doubted WOR's sincerity in the hiring of Gatling, understand that they have also been airing Jay Diamond, Grant's fellow hate show host who once called a Black woman "a Black bitch" over the air-waves of *WABC.* WOR has also done nothing to censure Grant for the December anti-East Indian rampage and chose Martin Luther King's birthday for airing Charles Murray. Happy Birthday, Martin.

Appendix 22

The DAILY CHALLENGE THURSDAY JANUARY 8, 1998

"Claire Shulman: The Real Catherine Of Braganza"

By James C. McIntosh

Members of a group called Friends Against Queen Catherine say that Queens Borough President Claire Shulman is trying to "shove the idea of a seven-story statue of a white slaving queen down the throats of the Black and Brown citizens of Queens."They say that Shulman has endured heated meetings, angry letters from her constituents and Queens community leaders but she has not abandoned the idea of paying homage to Catherine of Braganza.

One of the leaders of the group, Betty Dopson, says that "Catherine is the 17th Century obscurity whose husband named the Borough of Queens after her, the Borough of Brooklyn after himself and New York's island after the Duke who militarily took it from the Dutch, who had stolen it from the indigenous inhabitants in the first place."

Shulman has countered that the statue is "a gift" from the country of Portugal in honor of the woman for whom the borough is named. Shulman has also, in response to the demand of protesters, recently said that perhaps the statue could be built on private land instead of Port Authority property as originally planned. Rev. Charles Norris, another of the group's leaders, says. "That's not good enough. Catherine must go."

Shulman has pressed on with her plans, and many are asking "why?" One unnamed source says that "Shulman's obsession with this statue is that she is the spiritual heir of Catherine of Braganza." The source recounted the following similarities as a way of supporting his argument:

Catherine The Slave Queen

Long ago and far away, there lived a woman named Catherine who was born into the royal family of Portugal, the first European country to raid the continent of Africa in the European slave trade. After a brief attempt to marry her off to Louis XIV of France, her family married her into the British royalty. Part of her dowry was the colony of Brown people called Bombay. Catherine has been treated kindly by white historians mainly because of the scoundrels of her day to whom she might be compared. Because of her relative obscurity, she has, among white people, maintained a good reputation despite her habit of finding herself surrounded by bad people who met her royal custodial needs. One possible indicator of her odd reputation and alleged bad deeds is contained in Eric Williams' classic, Capitalism and Slavery.

Speaking of people forced into 10 years involuntary servitude (slavery) in Barbados, Williams writes: "The prisoners were granted in batches to favorite courtiers, who made handsome profits from the traffic in which it is alleged even the Queen shared." Despite such specific allegations of personally benefiting from the slave trade, her main historical significance, prior to Claire Shulman, had been the fact that she married King Charles II a man who returned monarchy to England after a brief and failed attempt at government by Parliament under a Lord protector named Oliver Cromwell. Charles was a man famous for his lecherous adultery, his custom of making servants approach him on bended knee and for first minting the famous coin called the "Guinea" that became the currency of the European/African slave trade. Guinea was one of the early names for the Continent of Africa, the land Charles and Catherine most ruthlessly exploited.

Under their royal sanction, The Company of Royal Adventurers was incorporated in 1663 and the Royal African Company was created in 1673 both for the purpose of monopolizing the trade in African prisoners (slaves). Ironically, this Queen has been said by those like Shulman who want to build a statue to her to have not been really white because she had an olive complexion. This complexion "was, of course, the result of the abundance of African blood that found its way into the Iberian Peninsula," including Portugal, her country of origin, on so many occasions, e.g. The Moors, Hannibal and the Carthaginians and others. But Catherine lived white, married white and benefited as a white, as people of color around the globe were exploited. It has been said by her supporters that she did not own a single slave. She didn't have to, because everything she needed ways in her husband's name. She and her husband were a team. Even her revisionist supporters admit that she was fiercely loyal to him despite his evil ways. She was paid well for it and lived lavishly in comparison to others because of that loyalty.

Her husband (with her loving support) laid the basis for slavery's expansion by granting trading (slaving) charters to companies in North Carolina, Delaware and Rhode Island. In order to pay a $80,000 debt he owed William Penn, the man who stole the island of Jamaica for England, he gave Penn's son a small plot of land belonging to the so-called Indians that later came to be known as the State of Pennsylvania. Charles developed another Slave capital by establishing Barbados as a Crown colony in 1663. Catherine slept and ate well as countless suffered at her monarchy's suppression of a major slave rebellion there in 1672. Also, many of the people in Catherine's own court at home, called servants were de facto slaves. These servants Charles had crawling around on their knees were certainly used by Catherine. It must also not be forgotten that every piece clothing, every morsel of food, every piece of jewelry she enjoyed was the result of Black misery.

CLAIRE'S MARRIAGE MADE IN HELL

Currently, in a place even less far away, there is another woman, named Claire Shulman who has come to power on a trail of blood and corruption staining the coattails upon which climbed. Those coattails belonged to Donald Manes the man whose name for many defines corrupt political machine. In this political analogy, Manes could be thought of as Claire's political father and the corrupt machine that spawned her is analogous to the slaving government that for political benefit gave/married/bought her into the court of New York. Good Boss Claire has just wed. No not that kind of wedding! She married a physician a long ago. Claire has just consummated a political marriage to the boss of the five boroughs, Rudy Giuliani, who is more than a little similar to King Charles II. Certainly, Rudolph has returned the monarchy to New York.

Just as Catherine's marriage was designed to bring peace and mutual benefit to historically military, religious and political enemies, Claire's marriage is meant to do the same. This is Claire's last term as Borough President. This is for Rudolph the last term he can serve as mayor. He needs to broaden his support as he attempts to move on to national office and fulfill his boyhood dream of becoming the first Italian American Catholic president. J.F. Kennedy was his model. Again the analogies bound. Claire on the other hand, can benefit by his support as she moves to become the boss of the five boroughs in the year 2001. And certainly there maybe bad blood between the two.

A QUEENS TALE: CLAIRE'S TRAIL OF BLOOD AND CORRUPTION

Eleven years ago, in the early spring of 1986, Claire's Boss and political father Donald Manes, died under what an only be called extremely unusual circumstances. He had a knife wound to the chest that punctured his heart. It. was ruled a suicide. The precipitant was thought to be the footsteps of an aggressive young counselor named Giuliani who from his office of U.S. attorney was literally muscling his way into New York politics by investigating and indicting every local politician that got in his way, including Bronx Democratic chair Stanley Friedman and Queens Borough President Donald Manes.

Two months before Manes killed himself in this unusual way he was found by police in a car with both wrists slashed so severely that he suffered a heart attack from blood loss. His original story was that he had been abducted and cut in this way by two strangers. One week after his abduction, Rudolph Giuliani's office used Manes convalescence period to announce that Manes was the target of a Parking Violations Department investigation. Four days after this announcement, under pressure from many quarters, political friends such as boss of the five boroughs, Mayor Edward Koch, the New York media, the Justice Department and other law enforcement officials, Manes changed his story to say he had inflicted the wounds himself

SWEEP THE BODIES UNDER MANES

In the context of this tremendous loss of credibility, a great deal of New York City's business-as-usual corruption got swept under the name of Donald Manes. The very next day after Manes changed his abduction story, a Queens attorney named Michael Dowd confessed to Federal prosecutors that Manes had extorted over $36,000 over an 18-month period. And within a week, the "Boss of The Five Boroughs," Ed Koch called his old friend Manes a crook and called for him to be jailed. During that "sweep the bodies under Manes period," local capos—called commissioners—fell like flies. But Koch was not touched. He, early on, became a part of the Giuliani political harem as would later Shulman, though she has not been as easy a date.("Andrew Gliedman, commissioner of HPD; Robert Litke, commissioner of General Services; Jay Turnoff Taxi and Limousine Commissioner; Lawrence Kieves Business Development Commissioner; Richard Rubin, Secretary of Queens County Democratic Party; all lost jobs under a cloud.

CLAIRE KNEW THE DEAL

Rubin had been the referee to oversee Shulman's mangement of the finances for an elderly woman named May Wagner. For doing this work, Clare had received $3,438 dollars in 1982, $2,349 in 1983 and was awarded $10,278 in 1984 (though this last fee she said she did not receive until 1985). She did not disclose these fees on her 1982 or 1984 financial disclosure forms to the city. Her 1983 financial disclosure form could not be found as of February 1986. When these things were brought to her attention in 1986, after Manes' resignation, Claire told a reporter "this would probably knock me out of the box" for obtaining permanent appointment as the Queens Borough President. But it did not. Both Koch and Donald Manes' deputy, Claire Shulman, though under a large cloud, did not fall. Rudolph apparently did not push hard against these future brides.

Few people believed that such corruption could abound around these two savvy politicians and they would not know. As Cathy Nolan, the Democratic assembly person from Ridgewood at the time, said: "If (Claire) didn't know, (she) should have." Shulman's rival for the office Lois Marbach, said it another way: "She knew or should have known."

INCEST AND BAD BLOOD

Even though Claire was spared by **Giuliani**, there was, for a long time and probably still is—bad blood between them. Many say Claire blamed Rudy for Manes' death. On March 3, 1993 in the security of the still sitting Dinkins' administration, Shulman may have taken her best shot at the mayor's weakest spot—no not Christina Lategano. She may not even have been around yet. That spot was Jim Hall. Few politicos had heard that name even in March 1993. But Shulman had. By special proclamation, she designated that day as Jim Hall Day. The occasion was the induction of Hall into The Black Hall Of Fame of Southern Queens Park Association. Receiving the award for this dead Black man, Hall, was a woman named Regina, described discreetly as Hall's "long time companion."

That woman, Regina, was also Giuliani's ex-wife and second cousin. That's right: Chinatown, wife and Cousin. Her father, Salvatore and Rudolph's father, are first cousins. She and Rudolph played in the summers as children at a home owned by Rudolph's grandmother. Because of Rudy's great influence, not much is written in the press about this incestuous skeleton in his closet (who needs federal prosecution and suicide by knife in the chest?).

TAKING THE SKELETONS OUT IN TIME FOR THE ELECTION

But for certain, she and Rudolph were married beginning in 1968. Their marriage lasted for many years until Rudolph got the marriage annulled, claiming he didn't know Regina was his second cousin. But the unknown source accessible only to the author says that "Rudolph knew, or should have known." Certainly, Claire's honoring of Jim Hall seemed designed to spark interest by the press in Rudy's skeleton in a period just before the mayoral election. Regina had, after leaving Rudy lived with Hall until his death in 1992. The unnamed source blames this embarrassing fact for Rudy's legendary affection for Black people. That affection has been demonstrated on numerous occasions such the time Giuliani gave standing ovation to Peter Del Debbio the white police officer who had already bee charged and was later convicted of pumping several bullets into the back of downed Black cop

CATHERINE AND CLAIRE THE RUTHLESS

It's not Christina Lategano, or his political marriage of convenience across political and religious differences that is Rudy's main similarity to Charles II. Nor is it simply Claire's recent (political) marriage to a despot that is analogous to Catherine of Braganza, It is both Rudy and Claire's deadly affection for Black people and their ruthlessness that is most analogous. Rudy is openly despotic but Claire is capable of smiling in a person's face then calling that person's employer to get the person fired. Claire is able, like Catherine, to keep an innocent public image while doing evil things. Recently, the cartoonist, Gantz, who first exposed Claire's seven-story monument to the African Holocaust in Newsday, announced that his cartoons will no longer appear in the paper. Members of the Friends Against Catherine point the finger at Shulman.

Chris Lehman, the "Currents Editor," of Newsday newspaper denies that Shulman had anything to do with Gantz's release from the paper, citing "budgetary reasons." Lehman further claimed that though he "understands that Shulman has been positioning herself in the Catherine of Braganza wars," he assured the public that "her influence does not extend to the editorial board of Newsday:' My source says she probably did. My unnamed source, accessible only to me, says: "Claire is as ruthless and culpable as the original
Catherine of Braganza,"

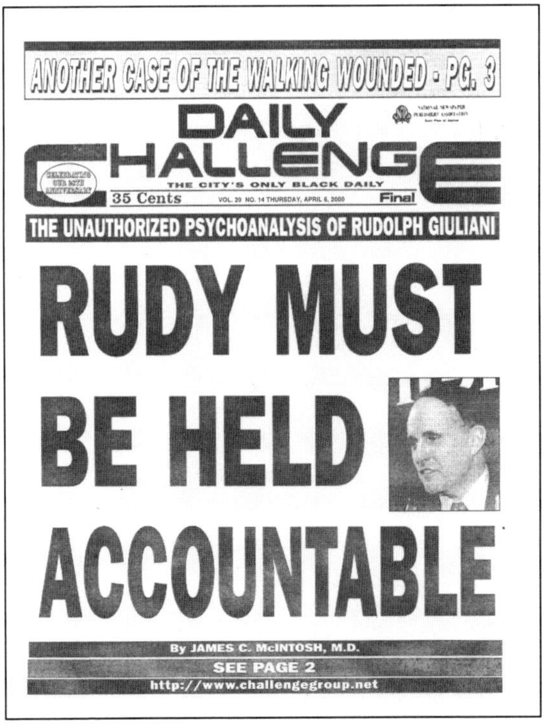

ANOTHER CASE OF THE WALKING WOUNDED - PG. 3

DAILY CHALLENGE

THE CITY'S ONLY BLACK DAILY

35 Cents VOL. 20 NO. 14 THURSDAY, APRIL 6, 2000 Final

THE UNAUTHORIZED PSYCHOANALYSIS OF RUDOLPH GIULIANI

RUDY MUST BE HELD ACCOUNTABLE

By JAMES C. McINTOSH, M.D.

SEE PAGE 2

http://www.challengegroup.net

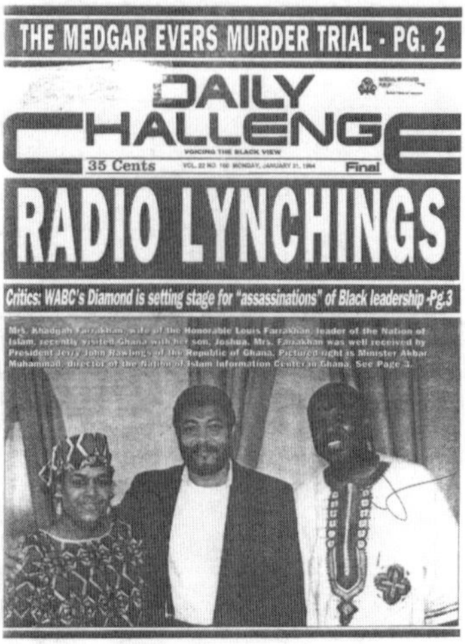

THE MEDGAR EVERS MURDER TRIAL - PG. 2

DAILY CHALLENGE

VOICING THE BLACK VIEW

35 Cents VOL. 22 NO. 160 MONDAY, JANUARY 31, 1994 Final

RADIO LYNCHINGS

Critics: WABC's Diamond is setting stage for "assassinations" of Black leadership -Pg.3

Mrs. Khadijah Farrakhan, wife of the Honorable Louis Farrakhan, leader of the Nation of Islam, recently visited Ghana with her son, Joshua. Mrs. Farrakhan was well received by President Jerry John Rawlings of the Republic of Ghana. Pictured right is Minister Akbar Muhammad, director of the Nation of Islam Information Center in Ghana. See Page 3.

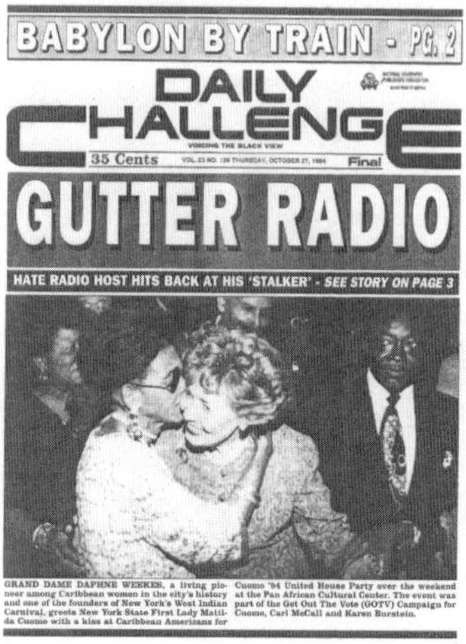

BABYLON BY TRAIN - PG. 2

DAILY CHALLENGE

VOICING THE BLACK VIEW

35 Cents VOL. 23 NO. 139 THURSDAY, OCTOBER 27, 1994 Final

GUTTER RADIO

HATE RADIO HOST HITS BACK AT HIS 'STALKER' - SEE STORY ON PAGE 3

GRAND DAME DAPHNE WEEKES, a living pioneer among Caribbean women in the city's history and one of the founders of New York's West Indian Carnival, greets New York State First Lady Matilda Cuomo with a kiss at Caribbean Americans for Cuomo '94 United House Party over the weekend at the Pan African Cultural Center. The event was part of the Get Out The Vote (GOTV) Campaign for Cuomo, Carl McCall and Karen Burstein.

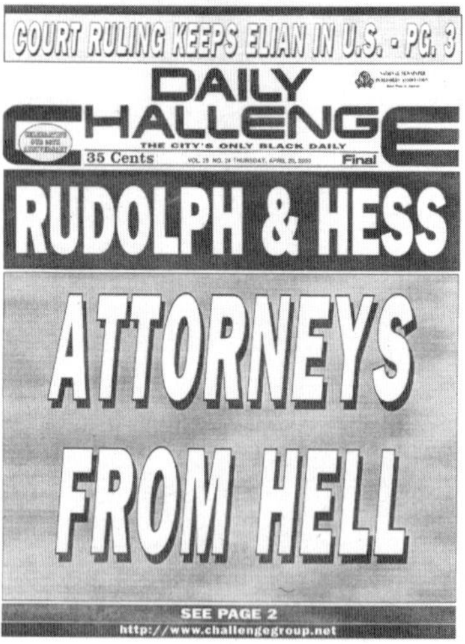

COURT RULING KEEPS ELIAN IN U.S. - PG. 3

DAILY CHALLENGE

THE CITY'S ONLY BLACK DAILY

35 Cents VOL. 29 NO. 24 THURSDAY, APRIL 20, 2000 Final

RUDOLPH & HESS

ATTORNEYS FROM HELL

SEE PAGE 2

http://www.challengegroup.net

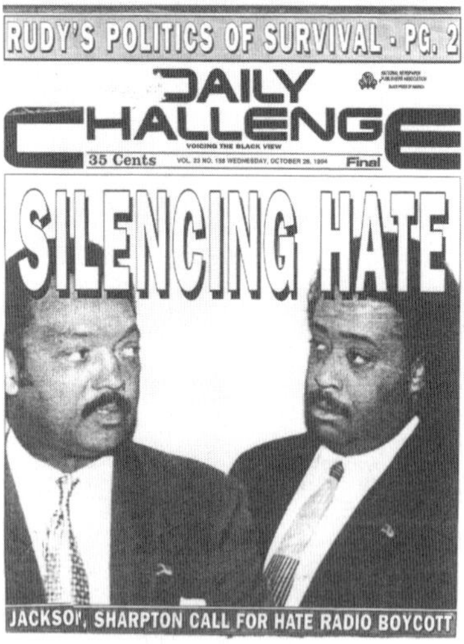

RUDY'S POLITICS OF SURVIVAL - PG. 2

DAILY CHALLENGE

VOICING THE BLACK VIEW

35 Cents VOL. 23 NO. 138 WEDNESDAY, OCTOBER 26, 1994 Final

SILENCING HATE

JACKSON, SHARPTON CALL FOR HATE RADIO BOYCOTT

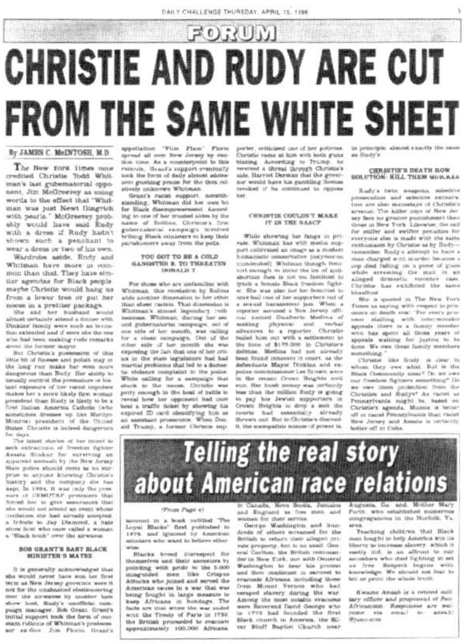

DAILY CHALLENGE THURSDAY, APRIL 15, 1999

FORUM

CHRISTIE AND RUDY ARE CUT FROM THE SAME WHITE SHEET

By JAMES C. McINTOSH, M.D.

TOU GOT TO BE A COLD GANGSTER B. TO THREATEN DONALD T

CHRISTIE COULDN'T MAKE IT IN THE NAACP

CHRISTIE'S DEATH ROW SOLUTION: KILL THEM QUICKER

BOB GRANT'S BABY BLACK MINISTER'S MAYBE

Telling the real story about American race relations

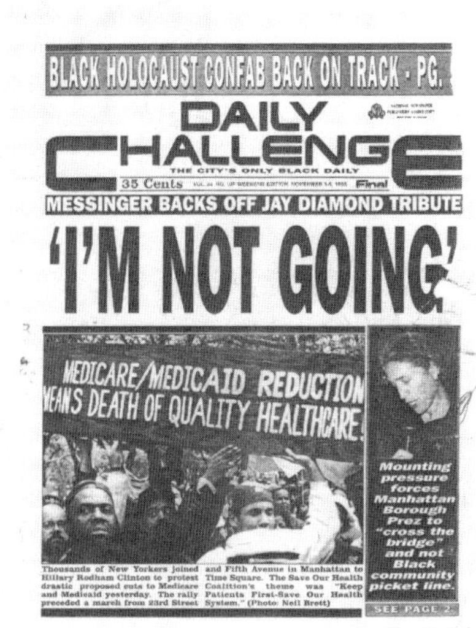

BLACK HOLOCAUST CONFAB BACK ON TRACK - PG.

DAILY CHALLENGE

THE CITY'S ONLY BLACK DAILY

35 Cents Final

MESSINGER BACKS OFF JAY DIAMOND TRIBUTE

'I'M NOT GOING'

Mounting pressure forces Manhattan Borough Prez to "cross the bridge" and not Black community picket line.

Thousands of New Yorkers joined Hillary Rodham Clinton to protest drastic proposed cuts to Medicare and Medicaid yesterday. The rally preceded a march from 23rd Street and Fifth Avenue in Manhattan to Times Square. The Save Our Health Coalition's theme was "Keep Patients First-Save Our Health System." (Photo: Neil Brett)

SEE PAGE 2

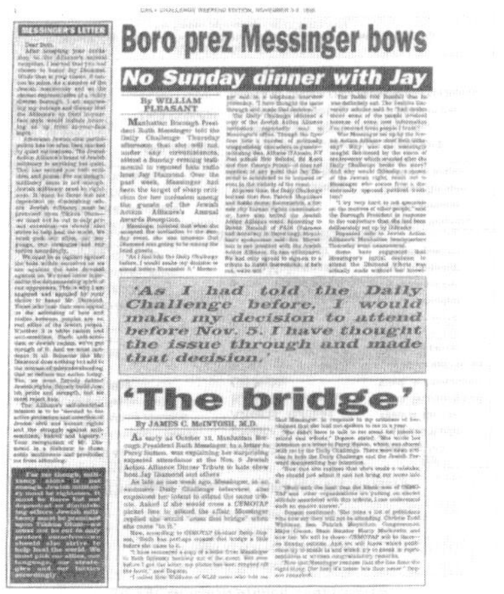

MESSINGER'S LETTER

Boro prez Messinger bows

No Sunday dinner with Jay

By WILLIAM PLEASANT

'As I had told the Daily Challenge before, I would make my decision to attend before Nov. 5. I have thought the issue through and made that decision.'

'The bridge'

By JAMES C. McINTOSH, M.D.

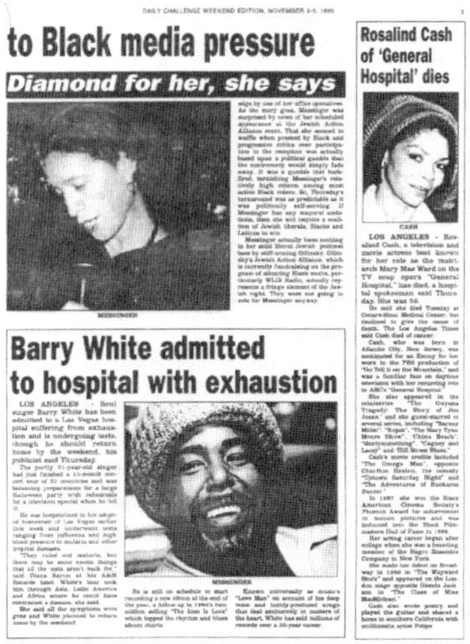

DAILY CHALLENGE WEEKEND EDITION, NOVEMBER 3-5, 1995

to Black media pressure

Diamond for her, she says

MESSINGER

Rosalind Cash of 'General Hospital' dies

CASH

Barry White admitted to hospital with exhaustion

MESSINGER

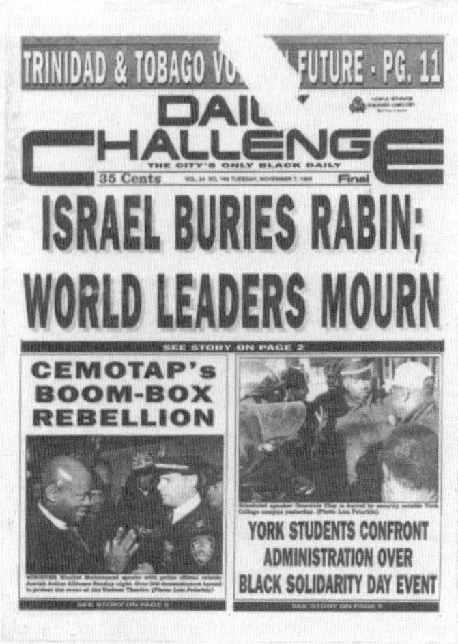

TRINIDAD & TOBAGO VO... FUTURE - PG. 11

DAILY CHALLENGE

THE CITY'S ONLY BLACK DAILY

35 Cents Final

ISRAEL BURIES RABIN; WORLD LEADERS MOURN

SEE STORY ON PAGE 2

CEMOTAP's BOOM-BOX REBELLION

SEE STORY ON PAGE 5

YORK STUDENTS CONFRONT ADMINISTRATION OVER BLACK SOLIDARITY DAY EVENT

SEE STORY ON PAGE 5

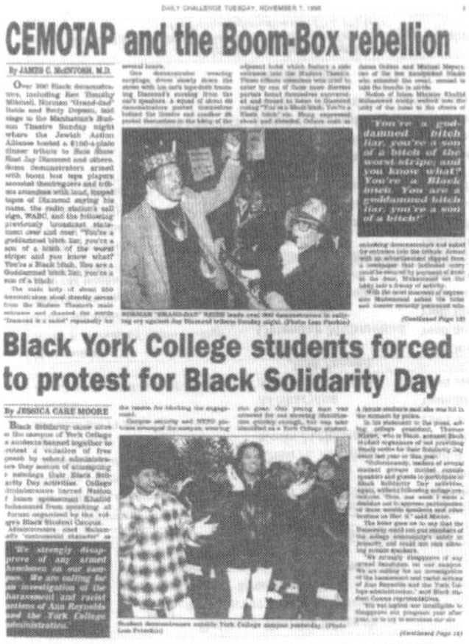

CEMOTAP and the Boom-Box rebellion

By JAMES C. McINTOSH, M.D.

You're a god-damned bitch liar, you're a son of a bitch of the worst stripe; and you know what? You're a Black bitch. You are a goddammed bitch liar, you're a son of a bitch!

Black York College students forced to protest for Black Solidarity Day

By JESSICA CARE MOORE

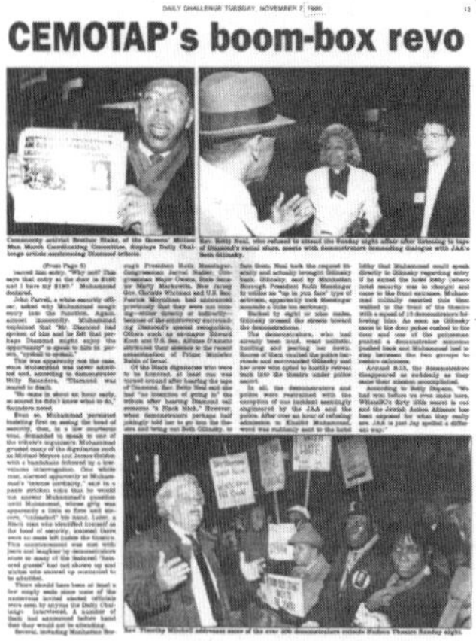

DAILY CHALLENGE TUESDAY, NOVEMBER 7, 1995

CEMOTAP's boom-box revo

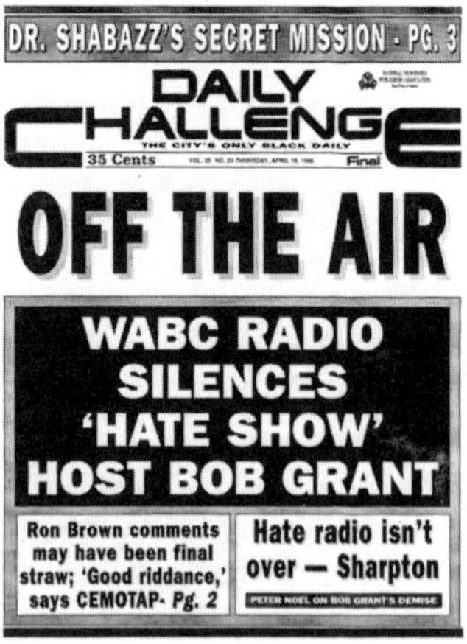

DR. SHABAZZ'S SECRET MISSION - PG. 3

DAILY CHALLENGE

THE CITY'S ONLY BLACK DAILY

35 Cents Final

OFF THE AIR

WABC RADIO SILENCES 'HATE SHOW' HOST BOB GRANT

Ron Brown comments may have been final straw; 'Good riddance,' says CEMOTAP- Pg. 2

Hate radio isn't over — Sharpton

PETER NOEL ON BOB GRANT'S DEMISE

Long before Don Imus came to the fore. CEMOTAP demonstrators linked hate radio to hate politicians and dumped Giuliani's "unofficial campaign manager" Bob Grant

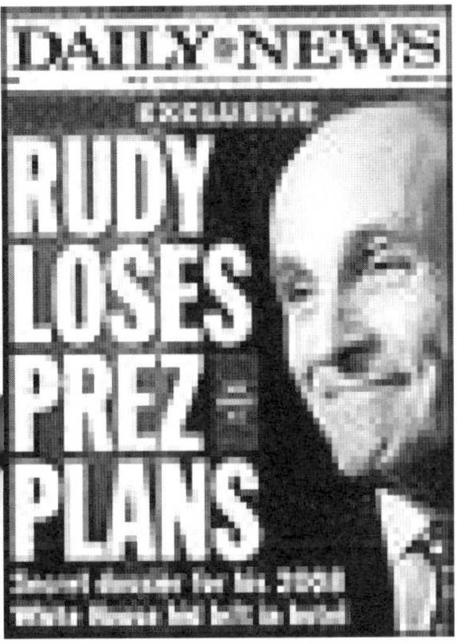
DAILY NEWS
EXCLUSIVE
RUDY LOSES PREZ PLANS

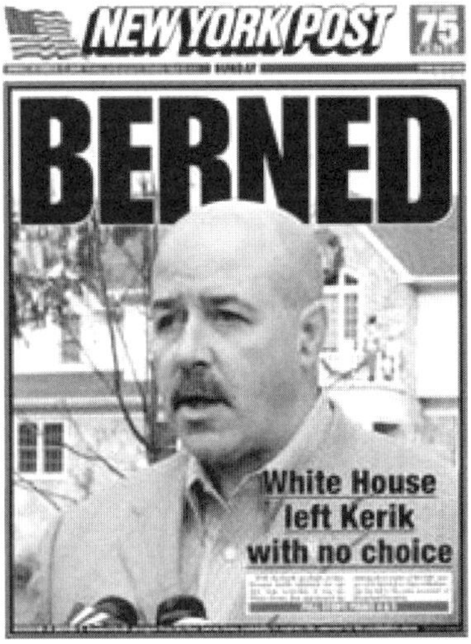
NEW YORK POST
BERNED
White House left Kerik with no choice

Since leaving the office of Mayor, Giuliani has developed a profitable relationship with Tazer International a company located in Scottsdale, Arizona that produces stun guns. His bosom buddy, Bernard Kerick ,who served under Giuliani as police chief and who was vigorously promoted by Giuliani as an excellent candidate to head Homeland Security has be accused and found guilty of fraud .

In 1988 Bernard Kerick was reported to be bankrupt, unable to meet required payments on a modest condominium in New Jersey. Today. The former beat cop is a multi-millionaire who serves as spokesperson for Tazer International.

Former NYPD chief Bernard Kerik pleads guilty

New York AP (Boston Globe)

Former police commissioner Bernard Kerik whose rise from beat cop to nominee for Homeland Security head was derailed by ethics questions dodged prison Friday in a plea bargain by admitting he took $165,000 in gifts from a company attempting to do business with the city. Kerik at a 10 minute hearing in state Supreme Court in the Bronx, pleaded guilty to a pair of misdemeanors under a deal that allows him to continue without interruption his new career as a security consultant in the Middle East. Kerik acknowledged accepting $165,000 in renovations on his Bronx apartment from a company attempting to land city contracts- Interstate Industrial Corp. a business reputedly linked to organized crime. And he admitted *failing to report a $28,000 loan from a real estate developer as required by city law.*

Is Giuliani qualified to be president of the United States? The decision is yours to make

Additional copies of this book can be obtained by contacting

Dr. James C. McIntosh
C/O CEMOTAP
135-05 Rockaway Boulevard
South Ozone Park New York, 11420
(718) 322-8454

Available books

That Which Cannot Be Destroyed
42 page broadside about the struggles of Master Mathematiciaan Dr. Abdulalim Shabazz as he trained directly and indirectly approximately half of the Black PhD Mathematicians in the U.S.

State Rape I and **Prosecutorial Misconduct** Two 40 page Broadsides about the related battle to secure justice in the Tawana Brawley Case falsely lableled a hoax by the media and the selective prosecution of a Black Charity, Hale House.

The War To Control The African Mind: A "How To Win " Manual 300 pages about the struggle of CEMOTAP for media justice and the larger global struggle for control of the African Mind.

Rap Music and Black Health: A Quantitative Analysis
128 pages about the impact of Rap Music on Black Health.

Dr. McIntosh is also available to discuss topics related to Health, Mental Health, Mental Illness, Media and Black History.

IMPORTANT NOTICE

CEMOTAP PUBLICATIONS IS A BUSINESS SOLEY OWNED BY DR. JAMES C. McINTOSH.

IT IS NOT TO BE CONFUSED WITH CEMOTAP INC.

THE NOT FOR PROFIT MEDIA ACTIVIST ORGANIZATION WHERE DR. JAMES McINTOSH AND BETTY DOPSON SERVE AS CO-CHAIRS

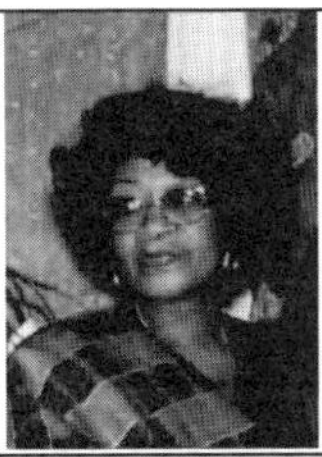	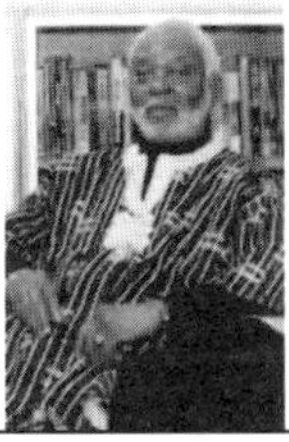	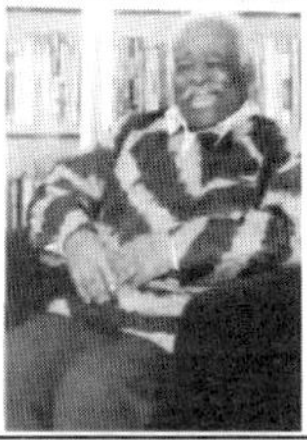
Suzanne Williams	**EdwardWard**	**John Pounds**
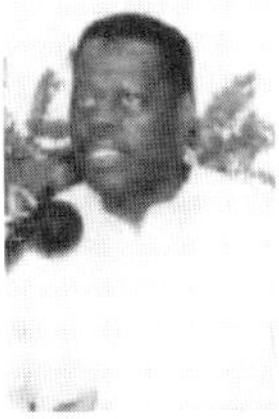	**EXECUTIVE COMMITTEE CEMOTAP INC 2007**	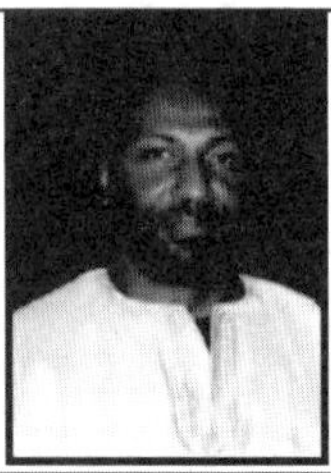
Bill Morgan		**James McIntosh**
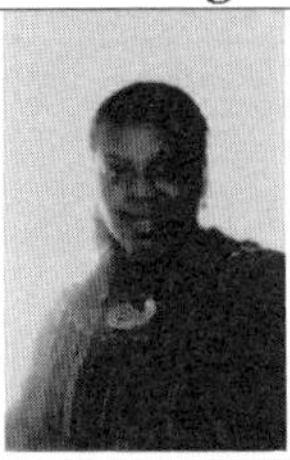	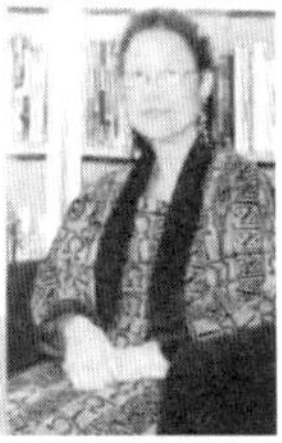	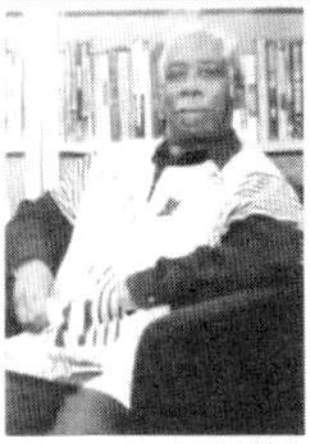
Sarah Mackey	**Yvonne Hill**	**Winston Greene**
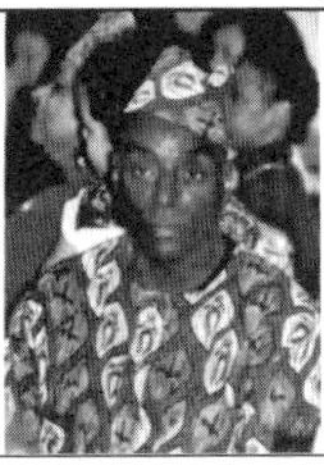	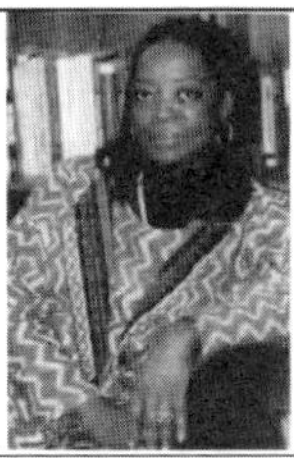	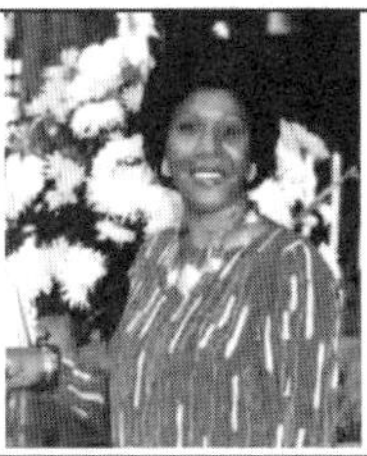
Ali Danladi	**Betty Dopson**	**Phyllis Cannon**

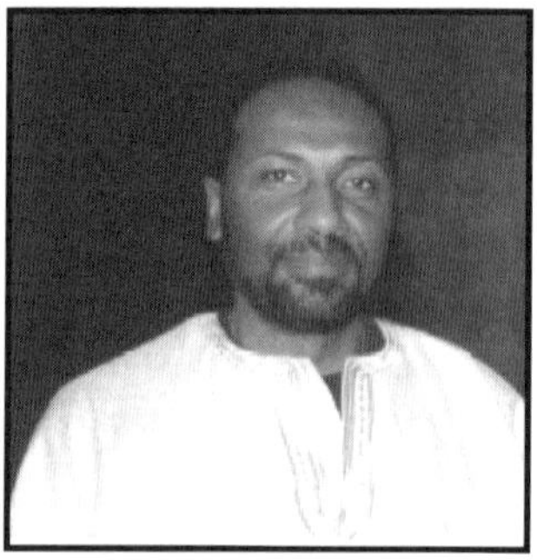

ABOUT THE AUTHOR

Dr. James C. McIntosh, is a Psychiatrist currently practicing in Queens, New York. He is the Co-Chair of CEMOTAP and a past president of The Committee of Interns and Residents (CIR), the largest union of salaried physicians in the country. He is a graduate of Brooklyn Technical High School, Hunter College of The City University of New York and New Jersey Medical School of the University of Medicine and Dentistry of New Jersey.

He completed 3 years of internship and residency in the Columbia University Psychiatry Program at Harlem Hospital. He also completed a joint year of Fellowship and Residency in Public and Community Psychiatry at Montefiore Hospital of Einstein Medical School of Yeshiva University. Dr. McIntosh was the founder and owner of The Interns and Residents Licensing Review School which operated successfully between 1987 and 1991.

He is a much sought after lecturer and the author of several books, including The Unauthorized Psychoanalysis of Rudolph Giuliani, That Which Cannot Be Destroyed, State Rape and Prosecutorial Misconduct. He currently writes for the CEMOTAP Drum .and is a former columnist for the Daily Challenge Newspaper, New York City's only Black Daily Newspaper. Dr. McIntosh served as Co-chair of the Queens Million Man March Coordinating Committee for the first Million Man March..

Dr. McIntosh has received awards from numerous community and Civic organizations and individuals including, The Bed Stuy School of Martial Arts, The Science Skills Center, Mosque Number 7 of the Nation of Islam, Women In Support of The Million Man March, The Coalition To Elect a Black Mayor, CEMOTAP, NAACP, United African Movement, Africans Helping Africans, New York City Councilman Charles Barron and 100 Blacks In Law Enforcement Who Care. Dr. McIntosh is a proud husband, father and grandfather. He is a past winner of Father of The Year Award from a coalition of organizations including The Southern Queens Park Association and The Queens Million Man March Coordinating Committee. In 2005, Dr. McIntosh was awarded The Malcolm X award from NAKO (National Association of Kawaida Organizations. Dr. McIntosh is an activist committed to the struggle for the liberation of African People and for justice on planet earth.